Grow Wild

THE WHOLE-CHILD, WHOLE-FAMILY NATURE-RICH GUIDE TO MOVING MORE

Katy Bowman

PROPRIOMETRICS PRESS

Printed in the United States of America

First Edition, Second Printing 2022
ISBN: 9781943370160
Library of Congress Control Number: 2021902155

Propriometrics Press: propriometricspress.com
Cover and Interior Design: Zsofi Koller, liltcreative.co

The information in this book should not be used for diagnosis or treatment, or as a substitute for professional medical care. Please consult with your health care provider prior to attempting any treatment on yourself or another individual.

Publisher's Cataloging-In-Publication Data
(Prepared by The Donohue Group, Inc.)

Names: Bowman, Katy, author.
Title: Grow wild : the whole-child, whole-family nature-rich guide to moving more
    / Katy Bowman.
Description: First edition. | [Carlsborg, Washington] : Propriometrics Press, 2021. | Includes
    bibliographical references and index.
Identifiers: ISBN 9781943370160 (paperback) | ISBN 9781943370177 (ebook)
Subjects: LCSH: Outdoor recreation for children--Health aspects. | Movement education. |
    Nature--Health aspects. | Sedentary behavior--Health aspects.
Classification: LCC GV191.63 .B69 2021 (print) | LCC GV191.63 (ebook) | DDC 796.083--dc23

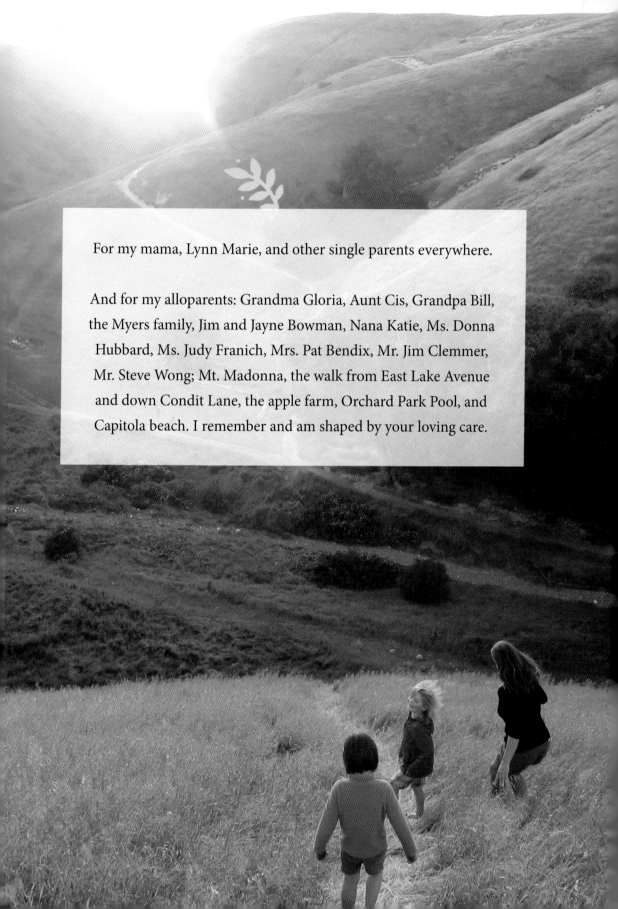

For my mama, Lynn Marie, and other single parents everywhere.

And for my alloparents: Grandma Gloria, Aunt Cis, Grandpa Bill, the Myers family, Jim and Jayne Bowman, Nana Katie, Ms. Donna Hubbard, Ms. Judy Franich, Mrs. Pat Bendix, Mr. Jim Clemmer, Mr. Steve Wong; Mt. Madonna, the walk from East Lake Avenue and down Condit Lane, the apple farm, Orchard Park Pool, and Capitola beach. I remember and am shaped by your loving care.

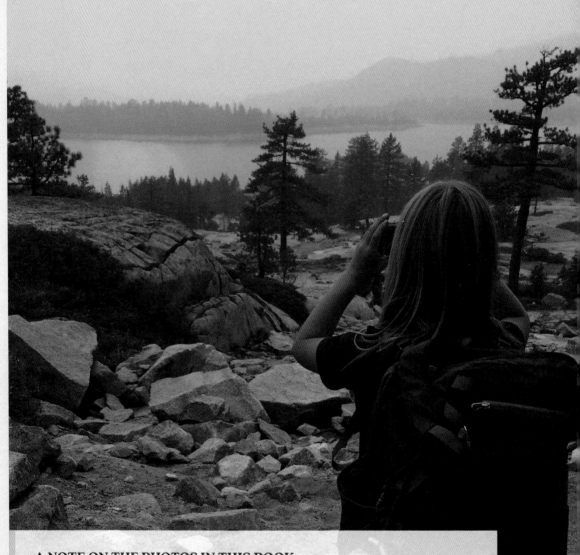

A NOTE ON THE PHOTOS IN THIS BOOK:

There are no stock images in this book; all images in *Grow Wild* have been taken by parents and alloparents (and sometimes children) as they live the ideas found in these pages. In addition to pulling heavily from my own family's image files, I asked my readers around the world to share pictures showing how they're applying *Grow Wild* principles to their unique life-styles and locations. I believe movement is for every body and worked to select a diverse range of photographs that show how different people in different places and situations are fitting more movement into their life.

Table of Contents

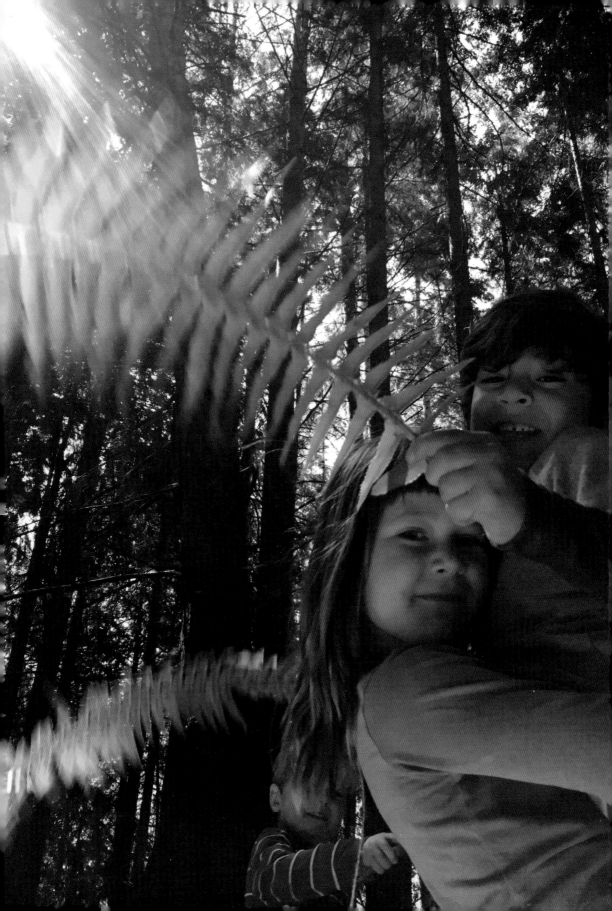

Introduction

Children are like trees. To understand how, let's start with trees.

From the moment they sprout, trees sense the loads that move them. Imagine trunks swaying back and forth in the wind, or branches bending under the weight of accumulated snow. Think of animals brushing past or landing on tree limbs. Think even of gravity, constantly pulling a tree toward the earth. All trees experience a set of movements—a set of loads—throughout their life. These movements bend and pull on the tree's cells, and in response, growing trees adapt their shape. This allows them to withstand their unique environment. A tree that is repeatedly pushed upon by winds will add mass and grow its roots in the direction and length it needs to thrive in the wind patterns it experiences. Trees in very snowy places respond to heavy snow loads by growing thicker branches. This ability of trees to sense their mechanical environment informs the shape they become and how physically resilient they will be.

Certainly, a tree's genes dictate its general appearance—oak trees always look like oak trees, and you'd never confuse a cedar tree for a maple. Its genes contain the information for the general shape of the leaves or orientation of the needles, as well as the bark color and texture and whether or not it peels each year. But the specifics of its shape are not dictated by genes. Genes do not control the exact diameter of a tree's trunk, the number or angle of its branches, the length and strength of its roots, or how many leaves each branch has. Instead, the tree's genes *direct its growth in response to the environment.* The genes say, "If you, an oak tree, experience X, you will respond with Y, just like other oak trees." These directions help the tree grow in certain ways based on what the tree experiences—movement, soil nutrients, sunlight, water, etc. All oak trees will respond oakily to their inputs, but because the inputs vary from tree to tree, even oak trees beside each other will take a different oaky shape. The shape of a tree's community affects a tree's shape!

Now imagine a tree growing up in a greenhouse—an indoor environment, where there are far fewer natural movements than outside. There's no wind, no snow, no animals nesting or climbing to stimulate a stronger shape. These sheltered plants never experience the loads that stimulate their ability to withstand forces of the world just beyond their greenhouse door. They become unable to survive outside.

Problems arise when you take these sedentary, indoor-raised trees outside into more complex environments. Now they suddenly experience loads that are much greater and more diverse than those they've been regularly exposed to. Outdoor plants grown inside are not well suited (read: shaped) to tolerating these different loads. In fact, in order to produce heartier plants, some commercial growers stroke (move!) their plants every day to simulate natural movement. They recommend not over-staking and tying trees when they're planted outdoors, so the trees get to experience and adapt to the movements in their new outside environment. This helps transplanted trees succeed in the long term.

It's also important to note that outdoor trees growing up inside don't really *flourish* there. They show telltale signs of living in an environment that doesn't fully meet their needs (for example, curled or discolored leaves, or spindly stems). Low sunlight, poor or excessive soil nutrients, crowding, lack of movement, unusual humidity, and a lack of other "outside" elements have predictable symptoms, even in trees cultivated to be kept inside. A frequent recommendation for raising healthy trees inside is to *get them outside often.*

Which brings us back to kids. As kids grow, they are shaped not exclusively by their genes, but also by how their genes respond to the inputs of their environment. Many inputs ultimately form a child, but perhaps none of these essential inputs—love, food, sleep—are as *constant* as movement. Our mechanical environment is moving us one hundred percent of the time. I wonder what shape the movements of modern environments are bending today's children into, and which environments will move them in the future.

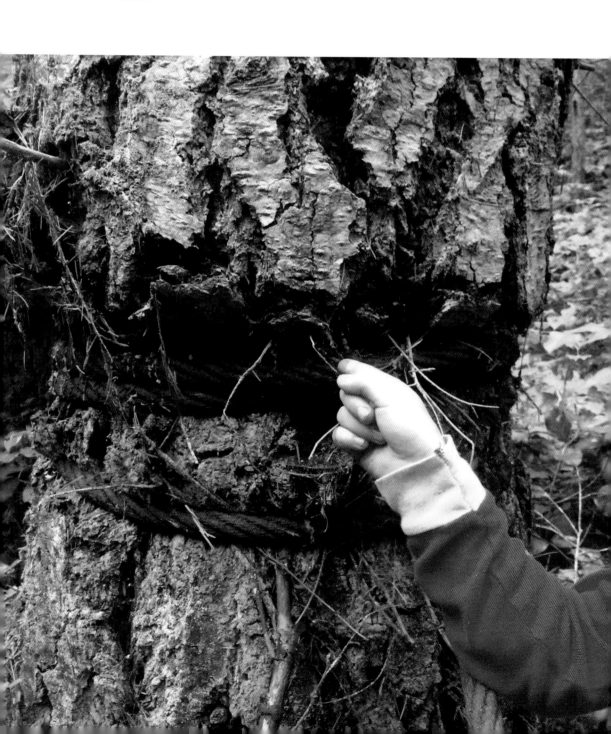

STUDY SESSION: TREES ARE LIKE CHILDREN

Biomechanics, my field of science, is the study of how mechanics (or mechanical laws) govern biological (living) things. All living things operate under a set of physical rules, so it shouldn't be a surprise to find that the way plants develop their strength and robustness is similar to how humans do.

The phenomenon of plants being shaped by how they're moved is called *thigmomorphogenesis: thig* means touch, *morph* means shape, *genesis* means grow. Nobody applies this word to the similar process of humans adjusting their shape to the loads they experience, but we could. If we had a word that quickly described how the way we're moved affects how our bodies develop, it would make it easier to see how movement matters.

I'm excited by the similar way both plants and animals survive in relationship with the earth (which is probably why I'm a biomechanist). As a human parent of younger humans, I take comfort in knowing there's an eons-old mechanism in place that allows for our best shape—we just need to move it. Children are like trees, but trees are also like children. Both grow in relationship with the mechanical environment around them.

Coutand, C. "Mechanosensing and Thigmomorphogenesis, a Physiological and Biomechanical Point of View." *Plant Science*, May 10, 2010.

Moulia, B., C. Coutand, and C. Lenne. "Posture Control and Skeletal Mechanical Acclimation in Terrestrial Plants: Implications for Mechanical Modeling of Plant Architecture." *American Journal of Botany*, October 2006.

MOVEMENT MATTERS

Total human movement is undergoing an exponential decline. If we represent the whole of human history with a single twenty-four-hour day, it took only one hour for anatomically modern humans to transition from hunting and gathering to farming, and a single minute for our culture to shift from farming to the Industrial Revolution to the Information Age. In mere seconds our bodies have gone from the dawn of computers to having computers that fit in our hands (and are in our hands for hours each day). Each of these technological steps forward was also a step toward decreased movement, but we are now in entirely new territory of rapidly accelerating sedentarism. This is true for all humans, but for the sake of this book and our species, I need to stress that **human children have never moved as little as they move today.**

Most people reading this grew up in an unprecedentedly sedentary culture, but in one generation we've lost a tremendous amount of the little movement we had left. Today's kids are more sedentary than their parents, and are living experiments of a *super-sedentary* culture. The status of "digital native" awarded to today's children is unwittingly packaged with its sister status, "sedentary native": a body born into a new landscape with almost no movement. Our kids are movement aliens.

How is so little movement possible when our bodies require so much of it to function well? It helps to consider what movement is and where movement used to fit into life.

Human movement is *any change in shape of the body*. In its most obvious form, movement is the lifting and bending of the arms and legs, and the rounding, straightening, and twisting of the spine. It's the takeoff and landing of a jump, the stiffening of cartwheeling arms, and the tightening of hands around a monkey bar.

Movements that are harder to see include the expansion and contraction of the heart, lungs, arteries, and veins. These coordinate their shape changes with those in the ribcage and abdomen as we breathe and work hard. Bones change shape slightly under compressive (think jumping) or bending (think picking up something heavy) loads. Our eye parts change shape when they shift between looking at something twenty inches and twenty feet away. Trees or monkey bars push into hand-skin as we climb, changing its shape and stimulating its cells to form a callus. These movements are impossible to see without special equipment.

Perhaps the most difficult movements to see, let alone imagine, are changes in shape that happen on a cellular level when we stay in the same position for hours at a time. Though the arms and legs aren't changing position and the heart and lung movements are small, our body's cells are moved nonetheless, even when we're still. They simply move into shapes that accommodate static positioning. "Being still" is an exercise program the body adapts to, and sitting has become the most practiced out of all the kid movements.

For almost the entire human timeline, movement has been woven into all aspects of humanity, beginning at birth. Eating, learning, dressing, playing, building, foraging, celebrating, and traveling all required changing your body position over and over again, in different ways. Movement was inseparable from human necessities; every task was accomplished through movement. Millennia after millennia, children's bodies grew up experiencing all-day, every-day movement via loads created by walking and being carried a variety of miles each day, squatting, sprinting, climbing, jumping, digging, gathering, play-hunting, carrying, hanging, and sitting and lying on hard ground. The bodies that resulted could withstand all the movement required to succeed in that environment once they became adults. It's a perfect biofeedback loop: the work required to meet your biological needs today creates a shape capable of continuing to do that work tomorrow.

Humans are excellent tinkerers, though, and over time we've fashioned a society stuffed with conveniences that save us movement. Consider how we get drinking water. Instead of the leg, arm, torso, heart, and lung motions that go into walking to source and gather water and then carry it home, a small turn of the wrist brings tap water right to us. Instead of using complex and abundant movements to search and dig for tubers, clean them, and then chew them a ton, today's kids take a few steps and reach to open the cupboard for applesauce in a disposable tube. Modern food, clothing, education, games, homes, and travel have become attainable with almost no movement of *our* bodies required. For many, life has become comparatively movement-free, and the children in this sedentary environment are growing up in the human equivalent of a force-free greenhouse.

But here's the problem we haven't been able to tinker our way out of: our bodies and basic biological needs are the *same* as those of our ancestors who moved all day, every day, for everything they needed. Our physiology still *requires* all those bends, flexes, loads, lifts, and jumps as we're growing; all we've eliminated is the environment that easily prompted us to move.

I assert that the vast amounts of stillness created by abundant convenience, technology, and indoorness (and the corresponding lack of outdoor/nature inputs) is a contributing factor to the majority of the health issues we and our children now face. Like greenhouse gardeners, we scramble to create numerous interventions to keep our bodies going in the face of the overwhelming effects of what is perhaps the most altered aspect of a human's environment: the mechanical one.

That all sounds pretty heavy, but the good news is that while most of us no longer perform the amount and types of movement our physiology needs, these movements are not extinct. Children and adults alike can get moving again, moving in all the ways that nourish and benefit our bodies, by making small changes to the way we set up our daily life. We have a big problem, yes, but we also have a simple, accessible solution. Our big problem might not be that complicated after all.

MODELING MATTERS

I was inspired to write a book on kids' movement a few years ago after witnessing my daughter, almost three years old, try a movement that she saw on the cover of a book sitting on the kitchen table. The image was of a young woman in the midst of climbing up an angled pole; she had only one hand and one foot touching the pole. My daughter studied the picture for about two minutes before she climbed onto the kitchen table (which we allow, even encourage, for reasons made clear in this book). The windowsill was beyond her reach, but she could fall in its direction and catch ahold of the ledge if she was okay with that moment of falling.

I watched her reach her arms toward the window, stretching as far as she could but falling just a few inches short despite her best efforts. Then she climbed down to measure how far she was short, looked back at the cover, climbed back on the table, and leaped from the table to the window, where she caught herself and hung by her fingertips.

That moment clarified for me the difference between teaching and modeling. The cover of that book did not instruct; the cover modeled. Humans have been moving in complex ways for millennia, reflexively copying the older and more skillful humans around them. It is only recently, in the almost entirely sedentary society we've created, that the idea of *teaching* movement has emerged.

ENVIRONMENT MATTERS

I've been teaching adult humans to move well for more than twenty years, but children's desire and potential to move are so reflexive, so innate, that teaching is not necessarily required. What *is* required is an environment that signals and permits movement.

Adults create and *are* the environments—the villagers, if you will—for humanity's collective offspring. That means we all, consciously or unconsciously, set the boundaries of movement for every human child (and future adult human) who passes through our space. So our spaces—the literal shape of them, the behaviors modeled within them, and the behaviors required of people within them—are also raising our children.

We've heard it takes a village to raise a child, but let's get more specific about what a village is made of. Certainly it's the community of humans that live there, but a village includes many other elements: the sky, the dwellings (and the furniture inside of them), what you wear as you're running around them, the rules (no running!), other animals, the plants, dirt, bugs, and microbes, and all the movements happening between and because of these parts. Each of the village's many elements lends itself to our childrearing each day, but there is more to life than a village. The nature surrounding each village, the "forest," if you will, is equally important. There has never been a village or villagers without a forest to raise them. You could say it takes a forest to raise a village.

I once read a lovely explanation about natural selection (the process by which groups of living things adapt to their environment) that went something like: "A solution doesn't have to be optimal to be favored; it just has to be better than the alternatives." Every movement in this book will increase some element of a natural load, but it doesn't have to be perfect. We're simply

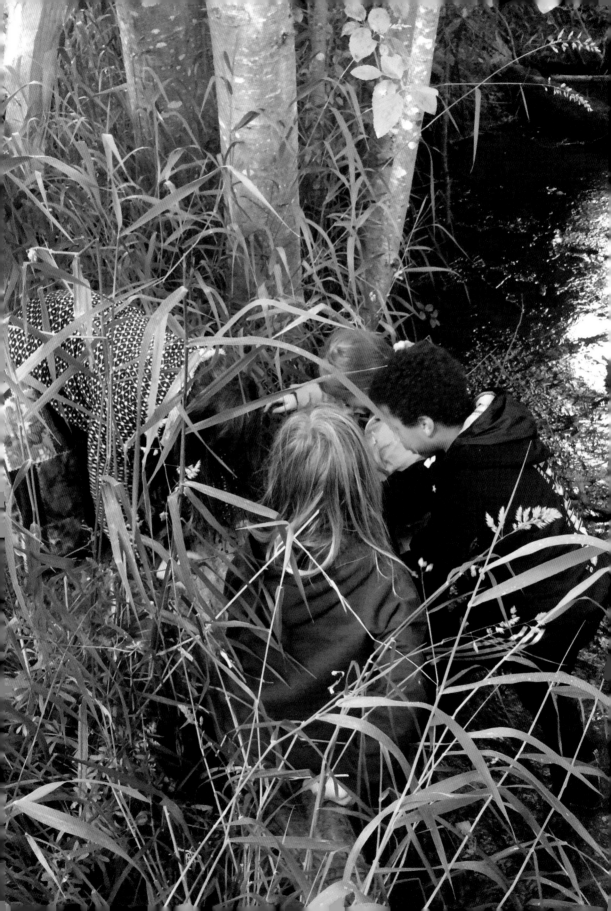

seeking ways of increasing the movement nutrition of our lives. If you don't have a village or a forest that is movement friendly and nurturing, please don't worry. The beautiful thing is that no matter what your life looks like now, you can find elements of movement, nature, and community described in this book and incorporate them into your existing home, routines, habits, and life. And you can meet new people, and you can plant trees. Even if everything is not available to you, something always is. Bodies don't come with all the movements they'll do, and no village and forest always existed; all are created over time.

USING THIS BOOK

Rather than being a book filled with exercises for kids, *Grow Wild* is a book about recognizing how sedentary culture inadvertently removes movement from our lives and how, once you see where movement used to fit into everyday activities and how it can also fit now, you can create space for movement in many aspects of a child's everyday life. I've organized this book by environment. You can read the chapter about the environment you want to fill with more movement to quickly find changes that feel easiest for you to make.

The environments are:

- The Culture Container
- The Clothing Container
- The Cooking Container

- The Home Container
- The Learning Container
- The Activities Container
- The Celebration Container

I've ordered the environments by, generally, the amount of time a child spends within them. But every family is unique: not all families travel; some play more sports, or do more crafts or music; some do none of the above. So their order of environments may differ, and anyway, the order isn't particularly important; the information is useable no matter what your family's list looks like.

Throughout the human timeline, most human movements were performed in a "green" setting and with a group of people sharing many aspects of daily life. Thus, I could add two other environments—nature and community—to the top of this list. But rather than tackling these environments individually by describing "how to get more movement in nature" and "how to get more movement in community," I've layered nature and community into the movement suggestions for all other environments. Moving more in the way *Grow Wild* explains will increase not only your physical activity but also your nature and community time.

Grow Wild is for any adult setting up an environment for kids—parent, grandparent, educator, therapist, sitter, or any other alloparent (non-parent providing care for kids). Children tend to model what they see, so these pages include photographs depicting all sorts of movement. And who says modeling is only for kids? A picture showing a simple way to set up a movement-rich celebration can get the "create-more-movement" juices flowing for adults too.

Grow Wild includes information about the science of movement, as well as what I'll call the science of sedentarism, but I'll focus more on practical solutions. We have more research than ever on the necessity and benefits of movement, yet we're *still* seeing decreases in total human movement. I'm not sure we need more facts at this point—we need to get the already-established facts moving. This book will help you identify both tangible and intangible barriers to movement, and it will provide a lot of ideas on how to remove them.

I've chosen to go photo-heavy and let each moment captured in a photo stand in for thousands of unnecessary words. Kids of any age can flip through this book and see others around their age moving in all sorts of ways, often on their own, no special equipment or even supervision needed. Seeing movements or movement spaces they might not have seen before informs them of the *possibility*.

MOVEMENT IS FOR EVERY BODY

Movement is for every body, but not all bodies move in the same ways. One of the reasons I've gone to such great lengths to define necessary and natural human movements as more than exercise is because when we make movement a huge category, it can include simple, nourishing solutions like *moving your dinnertime outside* and *moving yourself to school or work*. Humans and families come with a range of abilities, and while I'm not by

A SIDEBAR ABOUT SIDEBARS

This book is full of sidebars like this one, information that's separated out from the main text. We've styled all the sidebars the same, but you'll notice each has an icon letting you know what kind of sidebar it is. Here is the key for these symbols.

 Study Sessions: Digging into a book's reference section might feel daunting, but I've started you gently by highlighting an interesting study or research relevant to the chapter.

 Show and Tell: *Grow Wild* is not full of stock images; it's a quilt of sharing—parents and alloparents all over the world have sent in photos and stories about how they've changed their lives to get more movement. They have taken the time to share their experience with you!

 Movement Bias Check-In: We all have beliefs, and sometimes the most important exercise we can do is to look at them more closely and question where they come from. These sections are full of questions to consider alone, to talk over with your partners, and to use as diving boards so you can jump into deeper discussions with your family or other kid-related organizations.

 General sidebar: These contain information that complement the main text and read more like short essays. Some are contributions from other experts. Read them as you go, or flip to one for a quick bite or tip.

any means an expert in ability and disability, I've taught movement to a wide enough range of bodies to find that so far, adding more movement is always possible.

We're starting to see numerous professional therapies being moved into nature/outdoor settings. This is because occupational and physical therapies, adult daycares, and day camps for children can meet more of their patients' needs outside. You're not only receiving the benefits of the therapy, you're also being moved by the complexity of interacting with nature. If you're unsure how to adjust a section of this book to your special considerations, reach out to your healthcare team to see what insights they might have. You might be the person who exposes them to the idea that there's a more dynamic or nature-rich version of how they work, giving them the opportunity to increase the nature and movement for others as well as themselves.

MOVEMENT MATTERS TO EVERYONE

We are genuinely concerned for the humans of the future, and many are also rightly concerned about the forests of the future. *Grow Wild* demonstrates how the resiliency of both are entirely intertwined, literally and figuratively. They are bound together, as we all are, through movement.

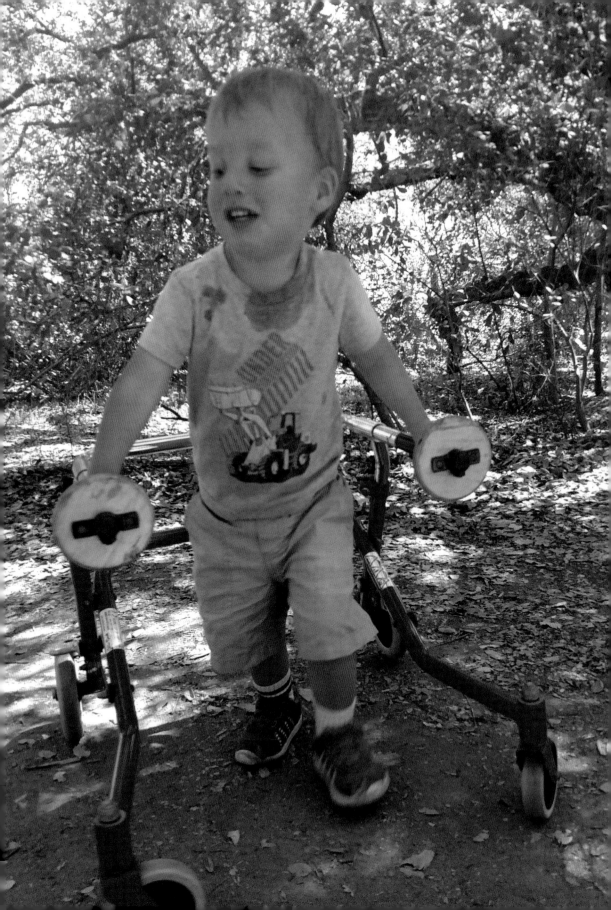

SHOW AND TELL

I am really passionate about helping my kids with varying abilities get out in nature! My husband and I live in California with our three boys, currently aged two, four, and six. Our four-year-old was diagnosed with hypotonia (decreased muscle tone) when he was seven months old. When Mason was two, he was strong enough to use a pediatric walker to assist him standing up, and he began to use it to walk independently, using the walker for support. We quickly learned that he had a thirst for hiking, often ditching the trail with his walker to explore off the path! We took his pediatric walker everywhere, and encouraged him to use it "off-roading" on the dirt, sand, rocky trails, and through puddles. His big brother was always his biggest cheerleader, and if Mason got stuck, he would help push him out of a ditch, or carry the walker when Mason grew tired and needed to be carried. We found easily accessible trails in our area that didn't involve steep inclines or stairs, as well as local walking trails meant for kids.

Moving together as a family early on has been one of the single biggest impacts on Mason's development. Now at four years old, he is walking independently and starting to learn how to run! I am so glad that we exposed him to the natural world early on, even if there was usually a lot of work involved for us as a family. We recently went on a family hike to a stream that was a two-mile round trip with lots of inclines. To see him working hard to power up the hills and experiencing the joy of being out in nature was beyond comparison. His pace may be different than our other kids', but as a family we all support each other and he feels loved and included when we enjoy nature together. I would encourage any family who has a child with mobility challenges to think about ways they can access nature together. It can take a lot of courage to start to explore the outside world with a differently abled child, but I can promise you it will be worth it!

—Ebey Sorenson

 PEDIATRIC THERAPY IN THE GREAT OUTDOORS

Laura Park Figueroa, MS, OTR/L is an occupational therapist and founder of Outdoor Kids Occupational Therapy in Berkeley, California. She shares a bit about her journey into moving her practice into nature and how she's helping other pediatric therapists do the same.

As children grow up more connected to technology and less connected to nature, a growing number of pediatric therapists from a variety of disciplines are exploring the benefits of taking their therapy work with children outdoors into nature.

There are good reasons for a movement toward nature-based therapy! A large body of research highlights nature's positive effects on children's mental well-being, physical development, and social skills. Nature offers therapeutic benefits that can't be replicated indoors. Spending time in nature may reduce anxiety and stress for both children *and* adults (whether therapists or parents and other caregivers). The sensory-rich outdoor environment invites us to move our bodies in complex ways while exploring with all our senses. Plus, nature settings often inspire feelings of awe, fascination, and connection with the living world around us.

Although pediatric therapists tend to see the potential value in nature-based therapy, they may be overwhelmed by the logistics of actually *doing* the therapy session in nature: *What kind of natural*

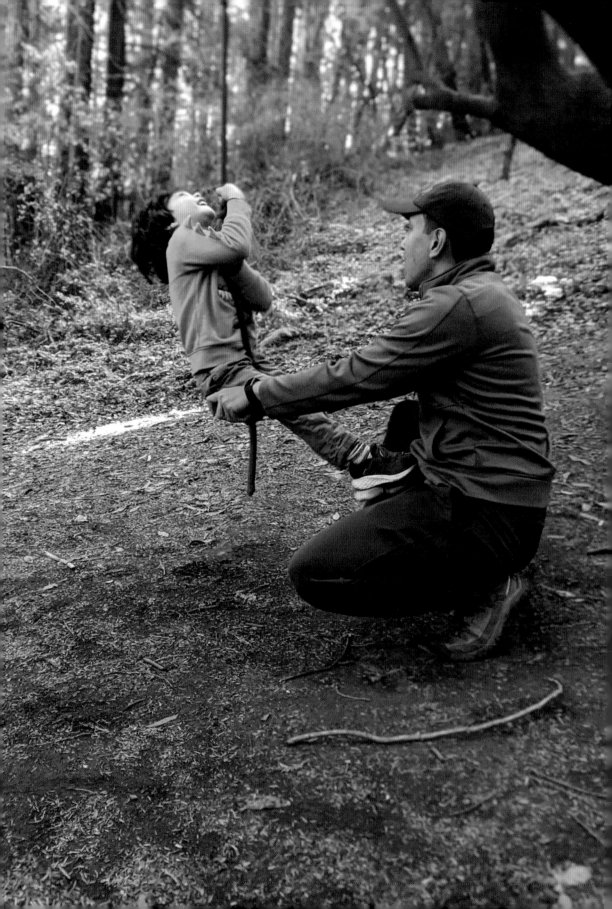

space is best? What will an outdoor session look like? What activities should we do? What safety precautions do we need to take? What supplies do we need?

These were some of my own questions when I started Outdoor Kids Occupational Therapy (OKOT), a nature-based pediatric practice. As an occupational therapist, my focus was helping children improve their sensory-motor and social skills for participation in the most important "occupation" of childhood: play! Nature seemed like the best place to do this work. At the time, I was unaware of any other nature-based therapy practice, so it was a little scary! I still remember my excitement the first time I invited two current clients to the forest of our local nature area to try doing an all-outdoors-in-nature therapy session. From that very first day, I knew I would never go back to working indoors with children!

The children were eager to explore and deeply engaged. I noticed right away how nature offered meaningful sensory-motor play opportunities. The children scrambled down an embankment to a creek, worked together to move a large log to make a bridge, and helped me set up a rope swing on a tree. To the children, it all felt like *play*! I saw the therapeutic benefits: multi-sensory processing, problem solving, physical exercise, risk taking, communication, motor planning, strength building, and social participation with peers. Along with these benefits for the children, I was refreshed being outdoors. I felt I was truly working in partnership with nature as a co-facilitator of therapy, as nature brought her own therapeutic value to the session along with my presence as the therapist.

Over the years at OKOT, perhaps the most important thing we've learned about nature-based therapy is that it's just like everyday life. Nature is uncontrollable, a bit wild, a little uncertain, and sometimes uncomfortable. It is ever-changing; every time we visit nature, the experience is different. This is in stark contrast to most indoor therapy sessions, where there is a tendency for us therapists to exert control over the environment to avoid any potential mishaps or challenges. Working in nature requires therapists to be flexible and stay curious during the therapeutic process. For children, nature-based sessions provide a safe space to learn to face some of the inevitable challenges we all experience in daily life. In nature, we all learn to go with the flow more, to accept things we cannot change, and to problem solve and adapt when things don't go as expected. Parents see their children's transformation into confident, resilient children with a deep connection to the world around them.

We developed the ConTiGO (**Con**nection & **T**ransformation **i**n the **G**reat **O**utdoors) Approach from our work at OKOT as a practice framework to help any pediatric therapist take their work with children out into nature. The ConTiGO Approach focuses on *connecting* children to nature and one another, while *transforming* their lives through evidence-based therapy in the immersive nature settings of the *great outdoors*. It is based on theories and research from the fields of occupational therapy, eco-psychology, and education. Parents can learn a bit more about our approach at outdoorkidsot.com and interested pediatric therapists are invited to join our free Facebook group Therapy in the Great Outdoors ~ Nature-Based Pediatric Therapists for support and resources to help you venture into nature-based therapy work with children.

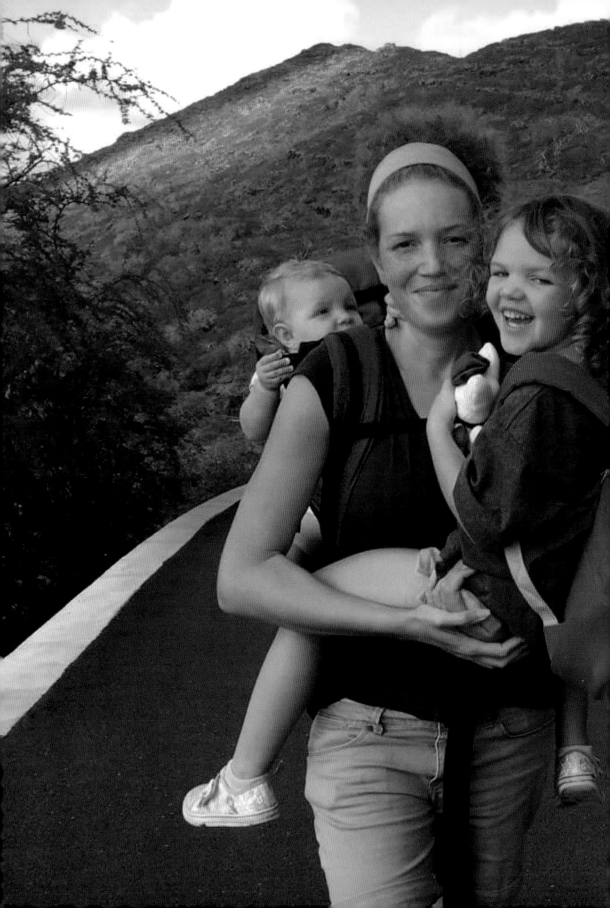

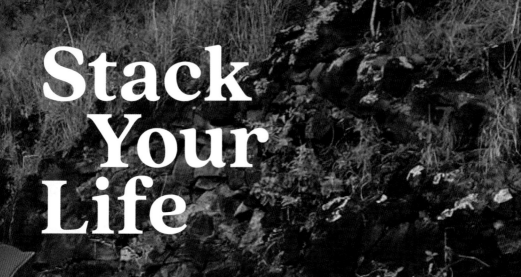

Stack Your Life

An approach to selecting daily activities so fewer tasks allow you to efficiently meet more of your needs and accomplish more, naturally. Example pictured: Walking to school (and/or carrying a kid as you do!), offers a variety of movements for you and them, family connection, outside time, and transportation all at once. See also movement permaculture.

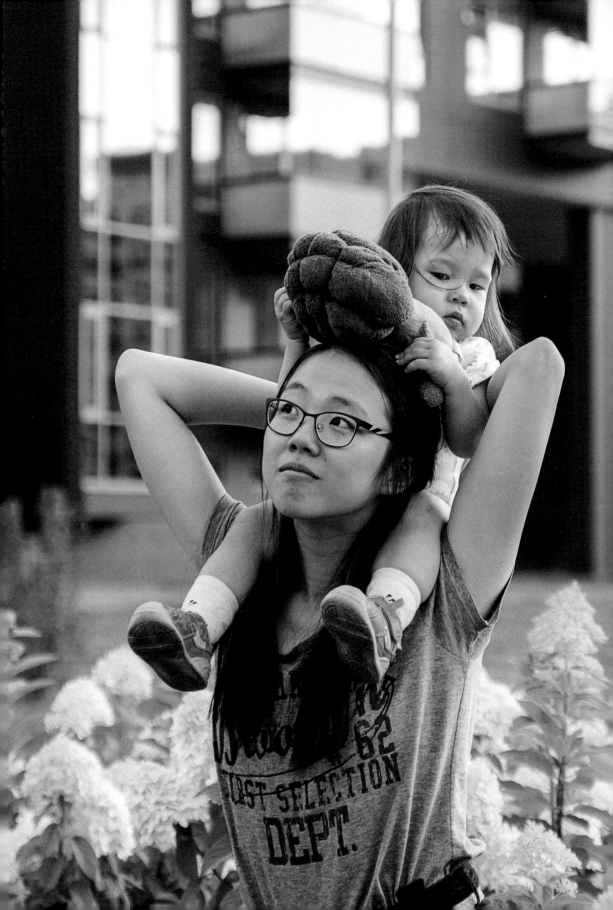

Stack Your Life For More Movement

chapter one

The key to moving more is *stacking your life*. Stacking your life is taking all of the categories of needs you have and, instead of trying to meet them one at a time, doing something that fulfills many needs at the same time.

I created the term "stack your life" before I knew much about permaculture—a technical approach to growing food that aims to save the grower's energy and time by setting up gardens and farms to mimic the way nature works as much as possible, making sure that each individual element addresses multiple needs.

MEETING MANY FAMILY NEEDS AT ONCE, THE WAY NATURE DOES

When I was a new mom, I found myself suddenly unable to fit in all the things that needed doing. And I'm not talking about the more fun, frivolous parts of my pre-kid life, but the basics: nourishing food, enough exercise to make me feel good, time to work/produce an income, and adequate rest. I couldn't figure out the biology of it all. How could having a family, an age-old human phenomenon, not align with me meeting my own physiological needs? As my kid got a little older and another one quickly came along, it got harder and harder to see how I could meet all of their needs too. The list of what kids need kept getting longer. Providing food and comfort was pretty straightforward, but they also need to move, learn, and play. They need peers, and peers of other ages. And nature! And, and, and. Forget about any needs I might have had; there was just not enough time.

After thinking and thinking about it, I came up with "stacking."

We all have *categories* of need. This list is likely not exhaustive, but I see the main categories all of us have as: WORK (both in and out of the home), FOOD, FAMILY, REST (sleep and downtime), PLAY (fun), COMMUNITY (friends, relationships), MOVEMENT, LEARNING (knowledge, personal growth), and NATURE.

Every day I wake up and know there are needs to meet. In addition to the tasks required for work (which seem to take up the biggest portion of hours per day) there are also those other must-dos on my list: have family time, educate my children, source nutritious food, move my body, move my kids' bodies, expose ourselves to nature—sunlight, the sounds of nature, temperature variations, etc.—and get adequate rest. Other category to-dos vary day by day (I feel less pressure to fit in friend- and fun-time daily), but all

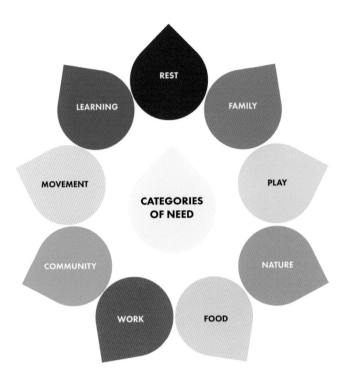

CATEGORIES OF NEED

categories of need sit at the front of my mind most of the time.

Each category of need could be met in a number of different ways, so I'm always choosing a *task* or *action* by which I'm getting what I need to do done. For example, a need for friend/community time could be met by a variety of tasks: getting together with a friend for coffee, sharing a weekly dinner with friends who have kids, arranging a play date for the kids, or a weekly session with a faith-based community. But some of those tasks meet the friend-need of only one person in the family. Others, like the play date, meet a child's need for community and their need for play. The two needs are stacked because they are both met at the same time by a single task. One of our favorite tasks is

Soup Night, where adults and kids gather in community to play, hang out, and eat. We often choose to eat outside (nature) and add a post-meal group walk too (movement). One task fulfills multiple needs of multiple people. Soup Nights are souper-stacked. Get it?

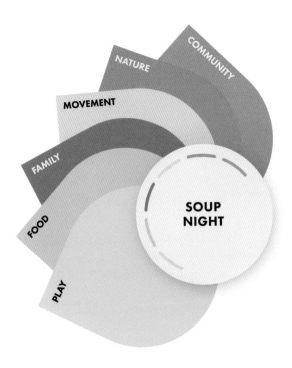

TASK: SOUP NIGHT
NEEDS MET: PLAY, FOOD, FAMILY,
MOVEMENT, NATURE, COMMUNITY

Right now, meeting your movement needs might mean different things for different family members. Maybe it's scheduling a trip to the gym for yourself for forty-five minutes, or taking a yoga class, or signing your kids up for dance or sports after school. Maybe it's simply booting everyone outside until dinnertime. Perhaps your infant's daily movement box is checked by "get twenty minutes of tummy time each day." However we are working to meet our categories of need, we typically select a single task and allot it some time.

I've had many excellent teachers and elders in my life, but hands down, the best instruction has come from nature itself. Nature wins for getting the most done for the longest time, and I've learned quite a bit about efficiency through observing natural systems. In nature, the "tasks" being performed don't happen one at a time, each requiring a separate amount of time. Nature meets many categories of need through very few tasks. Bees don't set out to get exercise or even to pollinate. Instead, simply by setting out to turn off their hunger signal each day, they simultaneously eat, keep their bodies moving, and keep their (and our!) food growing.

With bees in mind, I changed the way I thought about and scheduled my own life. Instead of breaking up my obligations and allotting time to each fractured need (i.e., twenty minutes to get food, forty-five minutes for some exercise, an hour to spend with my kids, four hours to produce something work-related), I realized the only way all my family's needs could be met was to find tasks that could meet multiple needs—so we could focus on fewer tasks while actually accomplishing more.

STACKING IS DIFFERENT FROM MULTITASKING

Stacking might seem like a new word for multitasking, but they're actually quite different.

Multitasking is making a list of all the tasks you need to get done and trying to accomplish as many of them as you can in a given period of time. You're trying to do *multiple tasks at once*, which is really to say you're rapidly switching between single tasks moment to moment and not really able to engage fully in anything you're doing.

Stacking your life is looking at the multiple needs you have and then figuring out a *single task* that fulfills many of those needs at once. Until recently, humans have been excellent stackers (like every other natural being), but modern society has separated everything from everything else. People live in small families instead of groups, school and work are done in different locations, we buy food in small packages hundreds and thousands of miles from its source, and movement doesn't seem to fit anywhere. At first it can be hard to stack our lives, because everyone we come into contact with is living in an unstacked way. Movement is especially challenging to stack— because nobody around us moves that much, we don't have any examples. Movement-rich tasks might feel weird at first because they're no longer common; movement has become counterculture. What binds us is that we're all in this sedentary boat together, which means we're all part of a group of folks struggling to meet our needs with the same unstacked tasks. We might not even know about tasks that can better meet our needs; our sedentary culture has forgotten about them! This is why I wrote this book. I've got a heap of simple tasks you can start using right away to meet your family's movement—and many other needs—at the same time.

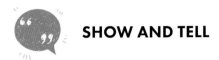

SHOW AND TELL

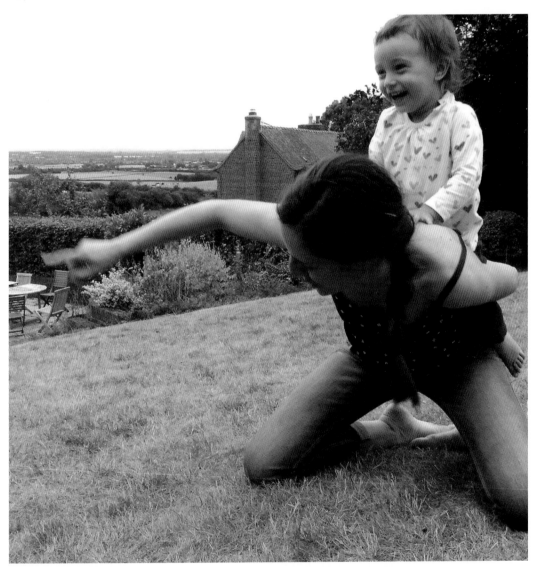

We are an ordinary family of three living in a small town in Italy. Before we become parents we used to be very active and spent as much time as possible outdoors, especially in the mountains. My husband was passionate about mountain biking and off-road running. When I was younger I used to climb and do caving, and when I moved to Italy I switched to swing dancing. Then we got our adorable daughter. And we were so tired that mountains started to seem too far away. We basically stopped. I suffered a lot because of this, got my self-pity period, and then I realized that even if I can't do my 10-hour hike, it doesn't mean we can't still enjoy outdoors and move.

My husband and I both have full-time jobs that require us to sit all day, so I decided that when I pick up my daughter from daycare in the afternoon we'll go for at least an hour to the local playground, and we usually spend this time barefoot on the grass and gravel. Works great in summer, but what about bad weather? No worries! I bought some rain clothes and we go play with mud and puddles.

I don't go to swing dancing parties anymore, but I have my little dance partner always ready for a twirl or two. And we have a vegetable garden! It's an urban municipal vegetable garden area and we have a forty-square-meter lot there. My favorite part of the week is when I have my free day from work and can go garden barefoot, listening to the birds and bees. It's four kilometers away from home, so I have a good [ride] there on my bike. And when we're at home one thing I appreciate a lot about having a kid is that I spend a ton of time on the floor. I used to do all my craft work on the floor, but playing with a toddler is totally a higher level of floor movement. It's hard work to shift the way I think about movement now when we have our little one and it's still a work in progress. We'll grow together and find more ways to feed ourselves wilderness and nature, I'm sure.

—Elena Stollova

STUDY SESSION: PHYSICAL ACTIVITY IN THE GARDEN

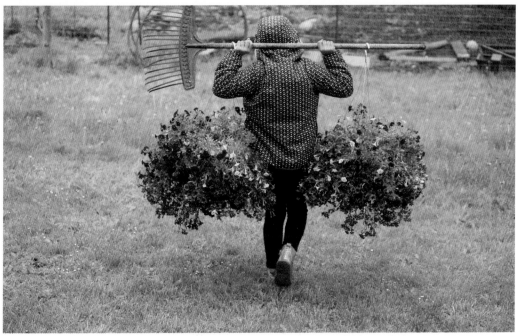

Physical activity is defined as "bodily movement that is produced by the contraction of skeletal muscle and that substantially increases energy expenditure." This means activities like human-powered transportation (walking, biking, or rolling a wheelchair to where you're going) and even housework make the cut. Gardening has long been a recommended activity for adults to stay active and mobile, but what about kids?

Researchers set out to measure whether seventeen kids aged eleven to thirteen also expended energy (calories) while getting their garden moves on. As you can imagine, digging and raking measured as highly intense, and weeding, hoeing, mulching, seed sowing, harvesting, watering, and planting were found to be moderately intense.

In short, gardening meets a child's need for physical activity and, as these researchers also point out, gardening is not only a way to get moving but is a task that adds hands-on experience in growing plants, maintains children's interest and curiosity, improves science achievement, and encourages better eating habits (eating more fruits and vegetables, YAY!).

Whether at home (family time) or in a group setting (community), gardening is a winning stack!

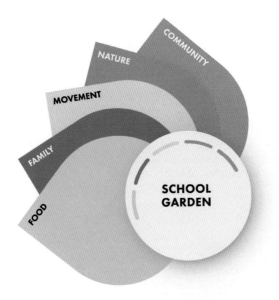

TASK: SCHOOL GARDEN
NEEDS MET: FOOD, FAMILY, MOVEMENT, NATURE, COMMUNITY

Caspersen, C.J., K.E. Powell, and G.M. Christenson. "Physical Activity, Exercise, and Physical Fitness: Definitions and Distinctions for Health-Related Research." *Public Health Reports*, 1985.

Park, S.A., H.S. Lee, K.S. Lee, K.C. Son, and C.A. Shoemaker. "The Metabolic Costs of Gardening Tasks in Children." *HortTechnology*, October 2013.

FILLING THE MOVEMENT CATEGORY

I think of every category of need as a nutrient. But consider our need for food. Meeting a calorie goal is not enough—our calories have to contain many types of nutrients in order to fully meet our needs. Food is made up of macronutrients, micronutrients, minerals, and vitamins, but all these terms mean is that there are elements beyond calories found in different foods that are essential, and in order to get all the nutrition we need, our diet has to include a variety of foods that each offer a bit of what we require.

Movement works the same way.

Nutritious movement diets, like diets of nutritious food, require a variety of nutrients—what I call *mechanical* nutrients. Kids' bodies—all bodies, really—need movement "calories," but they need more than a certain number of movement calories or "minutes of daily movement"; they need a diverse movement diet that includes specific movements of all of their body parts.

This is my way of saying that there's not a movement box to check off each day. Just like we can't just check "eat" but instead must make sure we eat a wide range of nutrients, we have multiple movement boxes to check in order to fully meet the body's need for movement-nourishment.

Before I thought through the idea of stacking, I found myself overwhelmed because I do not have the six extra hours in the day to facilitate what I consider to be essential tasks alongside the reality that I must work. Our bodies need a lot of movement, and we need to use a lot of our parts each day. I couldn't see how anyone in the family could spend as much time

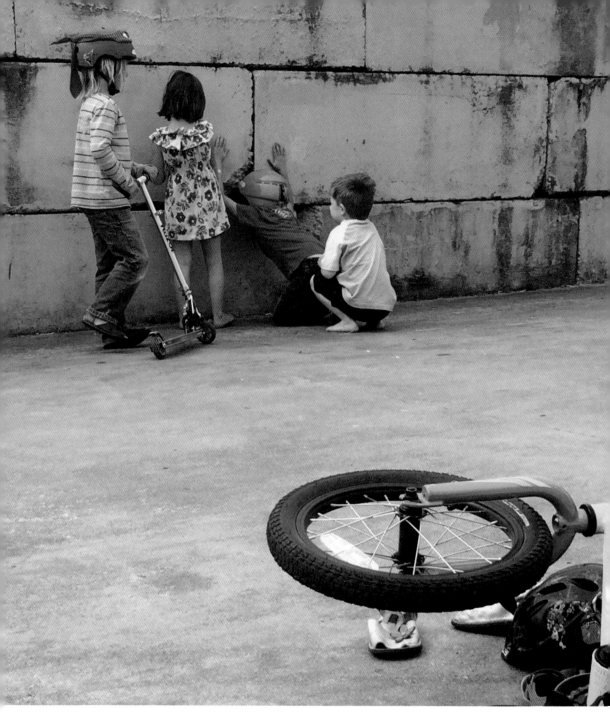

Nature is everywhere. Don't let the concrete convince you otherwise. This group heard some peeping and found a nest of baby birds in the walls of the skate park.

moving as we spent on our work or educational responsibilities. Movement, in fact, seemed to be the least important item on my to-do list despite being the biggest category of need. This is where nature came in.

As I noted earlier, most of the tasks earlier humans had to do to meet their needs required movement, were performed in nature, and were done alongside others. A simple foraged or gathered meal nourished the body far beyond the dietary nutrients its harvest contained; a meal might also include a group walk, conversation, plant-identification skills (nature education for the kids), and a body's bends, stretches, and squats. Talk about nutrient-dense! This is when it occurred to me: the "more nature" movement is also the "more movement" movement. More nature comes with more movement; less nature comes with less movement. If we want our kids to move more, they need to get a little wild.

STACKING AND MOVEMENT NUTRITION WORK TOGETHER

Research points to nature being an essential input, a nutrient just like food, movement, and rest, which is why I included it on my lists of needs on page 29. Our interaction with non-human elements has been coined "Vitamin Nature" by Richard Louv in his book *Last Child in the Woods*, in which he says that time spent in and interacting with nature is essential for humans, especially young ones. Our movement-free culture is also a nature-free culture, and this is not simply a coincidence; it is nature that gets all animals moving.

Our modern environments are, like our modern diets, lower in nutrients than their historical wild counterparts. Wild food contains a wide range of nutrients and tastes. Now our diets are made up of foods containing far fewer nutrients and tastes. We've focused on fast and pleasing foods, and now we can't tolerate much else.

Similarly, our movement diet used to contain hours of walking, bending, squatting, digging, reaching, pulling, and smaller movements of our body as it dealt with moisture, temperature, and the lumps and bumps of the earth. Now we've created physical environments that are very pleasant for our bodies—they have surfaces that are easier to move on, and they're cushioned and warmed (or cooled) so we don't have to move any body parts to adjust. We're simply not moved very much by our environments when we walk on flat and level (mostly indoor) surfaces, sit for hours in one position on our abundant furniture, and type and swipe on keyboards and screens. When you get rid of nature, you get rid of the diverse inputs it offers.

As a biomechanist studying human movement and how it relates to health and human development, I work to break down the *elements* of movement—specifically, the way natural environments move us, and how we replace these necessary movements when we're "out" of nature. From that perspective, let me explain how I interpreted the kid-craze of 2017: the fidget spinner. This transfixing spinner mesmerized many kids for a good portion of the year, showing up in classrooms, parks, and dinner tables alike. One thing seemed clear: kids were satiated by the sensation of this toy spinning in their hands.

MOVEMENT NUTRIENTS AND MOVEMENT HUNGER

Nutrients are inputs that our body needs and cannot work well without. Inside of the food we eat are chemical compounds (nutrients) that, when we take them into our body, create a series of chemical processes that affect how our cells behave. However, not all essential nutrients come from food: we don't *eat* sunlight, but when it hits our skin, it starts a series of chemical processes from there to our liver and kidneys and makes the nutrient we call vitamin D.

So how does that relate to movement? Movement has not been classified as a nutrient yet because we don't think of movement as chemical, but *the chemistry of movement* works a lot like food and sunlight. Through a process called mechanotransduction, the pushes and pulls of moving tissue also move the cells in that tissue. These cells convert their movement into chemical signals; mechanical inputs are also eventually chemical. So really, on the cellular level, movement works very similarly to food!

It's a similar story with deficiencies. Food nutrients were discovered and labeled as such because a) there are predictable symptoms that occur when their input is missing and b) the symptoms of deficiency are reversed when you add the nutrients back in. People first identified nutrients by looking at symptoms shared by populations who ate in a certain way and at which foods those people used as medicine.

Correspondingly, there are deficiencies that result from lack of movement. Movement reduces risk or improves the outcome for practically every physical ailment or diagnosis. Exercise science recommends bigger, "macro" categories of movement—cardio, strength,

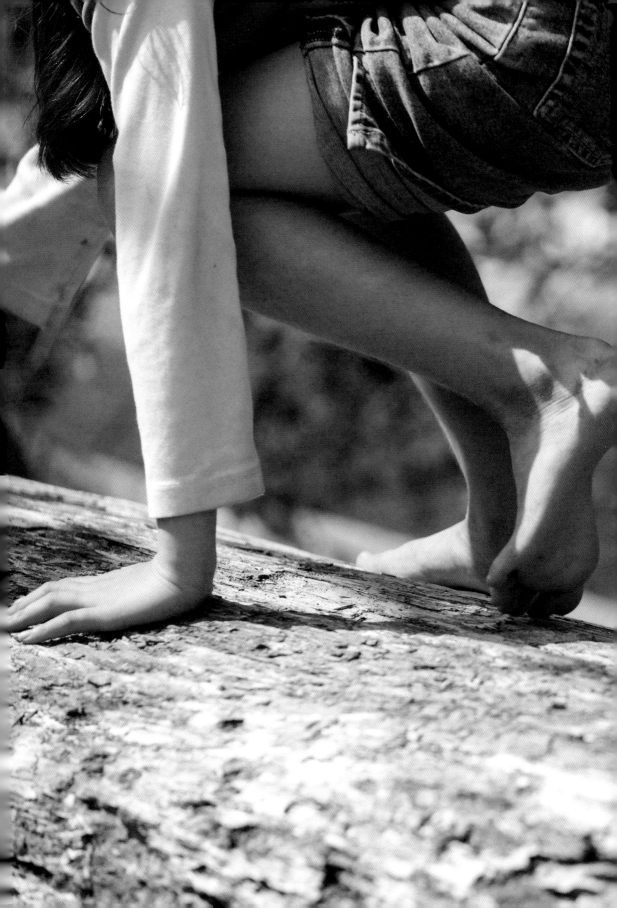

and flexibility—for general wellbeing, and physical therapists and occupational therapists regularly prescribe isolated micro-movements as medicine to improve the function of certain parts. We are already using a framework that is similar to food nutrient deficiencies, even if most people aren't yet using the same language.

If we viewed movement as a nutrient, it would be easier to recognize that issues that have begun to regularly arise and are labeled as broken physiology are really just predictable symptoms of multiple movement-nutrient deficiencies.

We know this applies to dietary nutrition. We know that the ache in the belly when we haven't eaten is a hunger pain. We can read the signs when our kids are hyperactive on sugar or cranky because they haven't eaten. We're comfortable with the fact that there are predictable physical problems that arise when we're missing certain dietary nutrients (raise your hand if you associate scurvy with a vitamin C deficit). But we are totally unpracticed in the language around and the signs of movement-nutrition deficiencies. Our under-moving culture is simply too sedentary to understand movement as well as our overeating culture understands food.

There's been about a five-hundred-year head start figuring out dietary nutrients, finding the macro- and micronutrients in food, and understanding why a balanced diet matters. We're just at the beginning of figuring out how movement works, but my hope is that we will capitalize on the framework we've already established for nutrition and add a baseline of movement and movement-types kids need, alongside the necessary proteins, fats, carbohydrates, vitamins, minerals, and sunlight!

WHAT IS NATURE, EXACTLY?

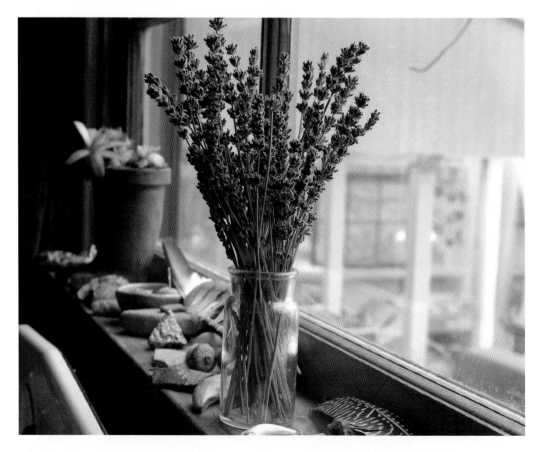

Humans have defined nature as everything in the universe except humans and human-made stuff. But really, humans and human-made stuff *are* part of nature, just as beavers and beaver-made stuff are. The reason we've recently found ourselves unable to deal with nature and its elements is probably that we've started thinking we don't belong in it.

Even though everything is nature, when we talk "nature," we typically conjure up an area or space that looks like what's often found in green spaces like wilderness, parks, and backyards. So in this book I, too, will use that more commonly held definition.

Wilderness is the least disrupted (most intact) version of nature we have on the planet, but you can find some elements of nature everywhere, even in areas that feel particularly nature-less. I've created a list of "nature elements" to help you see which are available to you *right now* in your own home and community.

- Varied temperature
- Natural light
- Textured surfaces to touch or walk upon (vs. smooth)
- Varied terrain (slopes vs. flat)
- Non-human animals (what others share your space?)
- Nature's artifacts: feathers, bones, shells, rocks
- Sounds (can you hear birds chirping, wind, bugs?)
- Plants (inside and outside, how much plant-life do you see?)
- Phytochemicals in the air (chemicals given off by plants)
- Smells
- Moisture
- Wind
- Dirt
- Bacteria
- The moon (daytime and night viewing!)
- Distance (to look to or walk)

This list is not complete. I have left out many elements, including non-tangible elements of nature like "hunger" and behaviors like "communication." But starting with this list, you should be able to quickly tune in to the "Vitamin Nature" that is always surrounding us and is always available for stacking.

I saw this as a result of underused hands. Compared to other parts, hands have a complex anatomy that facilitates diverse movements. From subtle movements at the skin and nerve level, to fine motor skills (like button-ing a shirt or grasping a pencil) to the larger-force grasping, hanging, and swinging motions that have shaped our anatomy, hand strength and skill has always been important for humans! But these days, the bulk of our hands' movements are reduced to writing with one hand, typing, and swiping. With such a wide gap between what human hands can do and what they are doing, children are missing abundant and diverse hand-activity. It's no wonder they gravitated toward something to keep their under-moved hands stimulated; *fidget spinners, like a candy bar, are instant movement-calories for starving hands.*

My kid will have me say here that fidget spinners are great. He found out he could create a breeze by fidget-spinning next to a candle flame. This evolved into experiments in fluid dynamics, which opened discussions on phenomena like weather and the invisible yet tangible forces of nature.

Fidget spinners also offer balance practice, observation and response, sensory stimulation, and in the way we used it with the candle, learning. But while the fidget spinner provides these nutrients, it meets them in the same way a vitamin tablet meets one or two dietary needs at a time. Mineral and vitamin supplements are one way to approach dietary deficiencies, but this approach doesn't often get to the root of the problem: not eating in a way that meets your physiological needs.

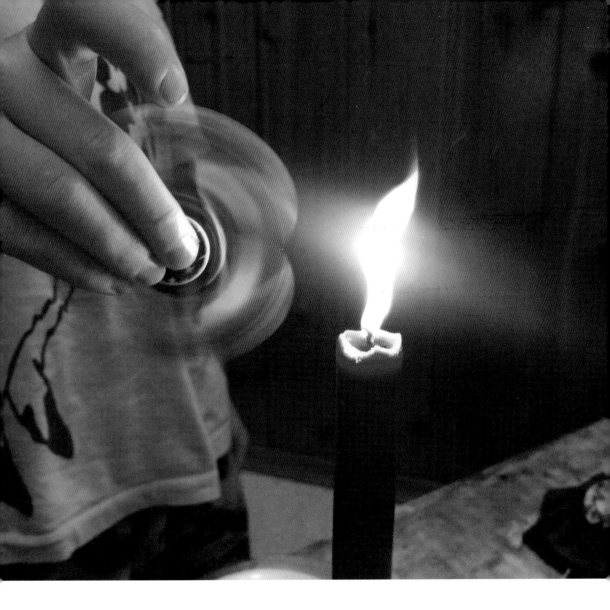

If you're hungry, you can eat a candy bar. A candy bar is nutrient-poor but calorie-dense, and it can still shut off a hunger signal. Why don't we live on candy bars, then? Because we need the other nutrients for our body to work. What if we thought of a fidget spinner as a candy bar for the hands? And if fidget spinners are simply an easy way to shut off the "Hey, I need to move and explore the world!" alarm in our hands, is there a way to turn off the alarm that's more nutrient-dense?

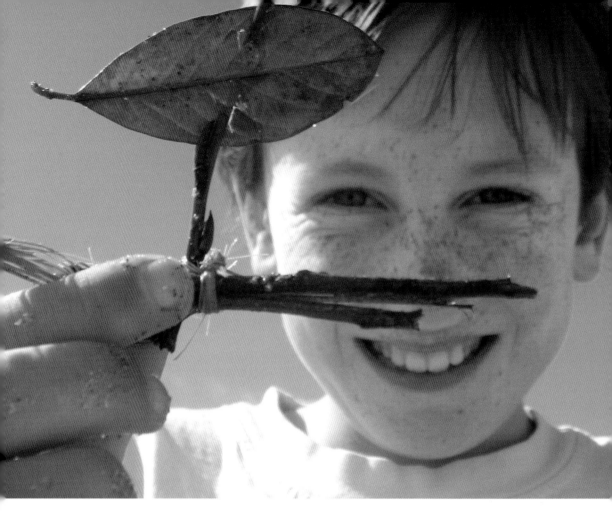

Nutrient-dense food is most often whole food—it's minimally processed and often looks pretty close to how it looks at its source. Nutrient-dense movements are similar—they are the "whole movements" humans have relied on throughout our history, movements that *simultaneously* provide us with shelter, food, clothing, and anything else we need to successfully interact with the natural world around us. Nature's fidget spinners, then, could be those motions that not only require mindful movement of our hands and brain, but also deliver experiential knowledge of how nature works and/or get us something we need.

One pursuit of understanding natural phenomena is the scientific method, and another is the sensory experience of nature in, around, and beneath your hands. Think of these tasks that stack nature experience with hand-movement:

- Catching and gently holding bugs
- Selecting and picking good reeds for weaving
- Weaving baskets and mats
- Making yarn and knitting with it, making cordage
- Picking flowers, arranging bouquets
- Tossing a maple tree's "helicopter" seeds
- Holding frogs
- Feeding birds by hand
- Foraging
- Digging in sand, mud
- Planting (especially with sticks or other tools)
- Gathering (nuts, berries, acorns, nettle)
- Processing gathered food (cracking nuts, mashing with mortar and pestle)
- Climbing trees

Each of these can feed the movement hunger that makes a kid crave a fidget spinner, while also providing a *ton* of other movements and benefits, including firsthand knowledge, skill, compassion, accomplishment, and a deepened and broadened connection with nature.

Each of these is also a task—just like "play with fidget spinner." By switching the task you use to meet your play needs from fidget spinner to any of the above (or something similar you can come up with!) you'll be meeting the "fidget needs" of kids' hands in a more stacked, "nutrient-rich" way.

STACKING IS CROSS-TRAINING FOR EVEN MORE MOVEMENT

Each body part has its own work to do. When athletes and fitness-folks vary their workouts to move more body parts, they call it cross-training. But we need to do way more "cross-training" than just a few different exercises, activities, or sports—we need to hugely increase our daily movement while also making sure the movement we're getting is moving the various parts of our body well.

I could rewrite the "moves for your hands" list for feet, arms, legs, and trunk. I could make a list of "balance-increasing moves" or "hanging/swinging skills." But one of the reasons today's kids (and their families) are moving less is because we no longer see the purpose of movement beyond doing it to be healthy. If we can regain that greater purpose of movement—to find shelter, get food, make the things we need—it will endure when we grow out of childhood. If we want to move more as a culture and as a species, we need to embrace *movement permaculture*, a.k.a. stacking movement back into our lives through practical, dynamic tasks that have been used by humans for millennia.

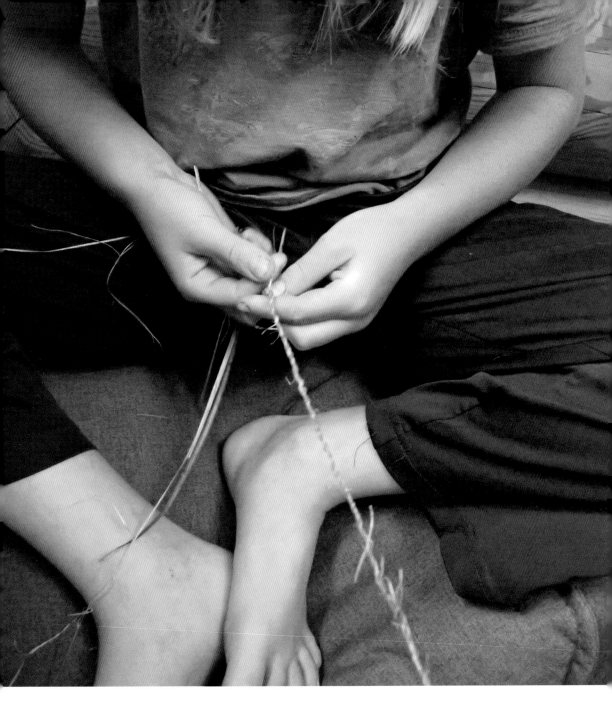

Cordage is nature's fidget spinner. Cordage can get everyone outside hunting for materials (we most often use trailing blackberry vines because they're abundant where we live) and identifying plants, and then it gets your fine-motor and making moves going. What a stack!

There are many cordage tutorials online to get you started.

BALANCING THE SPINNER

Just as we don't want our kids eating only junk food, we can also be mindful of the various "nutrients" found in movement. I can steer my kids away from junk food by offering them a wide range of nutritious food, and

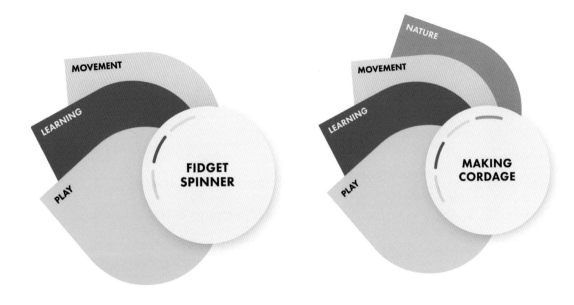

TASK: FIDGET SPINNER
NEEDS MET: PLAY, LEARNING, MOVEMENT

TASK: MAKING CORDAGE
NEEDS MET: PLAY, LEARNING, MOVEMENT, NATURE

similarly, I can steer my kids away from the couch by providing a wide array of nutritious movement options. This means regularly serving them time in nature or green spaces, and creating or finding tasks that require movement to complete but aren't necessarily movement-themed—tasks that help kids become physically robust and responsible for their own needs. Compare "Let's go get some berries for dessert" with "Let's take a walk for exercise." Same miles walked, but one task has a purpose beyond fitness and, with the reaching, squatting, and bending involved, a greater amount and range of movement.

ON WALKING

Walking is one of the most mechanical-nutrient-dense movements available. Walking uses many body parts, the "pumping" action of our legs helps circulate blood and lymph through our bodies, and the impact of our feet hitting the ground assists our bones and our brain. Until very recently, humans (as a group) have always walked a lot, and walking is part of why humans came to be shaped the way we are. Walking is also one of the simplest ways to get a lot of movement (it's free and you don't need any equipment!) and the most practical: if you're looking to move more while also getting non-movement tasks done each day, your movement has to be able to travel.

While families will adapt this advice to their unique situations and abilities, I suggest you and your family walk (and/or roll a wheelchair!) more. I suggest walking to the store and walking school busses, and walking play dates and walking birthday parties (don't roll your eyes until you've tried it) for those who are able. I, and all the experts and researchers of movement, have been saying folks need to walk more, but humans still aren't doing so. We keep walking less. This is why I'm going to stop saying "walk more" and instead show you how stacking this particular movement back into most other parts of your life is likely the key to you getting more of the experiences you've been looking for.

STACKING...IT'S ABOUT TIME

This book is about moving more, so the stacks I offer always have a "get more movement" objective, just as permaculture garden stacks always have a "get more food" objective. But stacking is not only about producing more; stacking is about wasting less. By choosing more nutrient-dense tasks, you end up consuming fewer materials (stuff harvested from the earth that quickly becomes our garbage) and you waste less time. You won't miss as many opportunities to get the basics you need. Stacking your life is not only a way to fit in more movement—as you'll quickly come to see, it's a way of *increasing the nutrient-density of a period of time*. This is what I love about stacking. Stacking is how you *increase the nutrient-density of your life*, naturally.

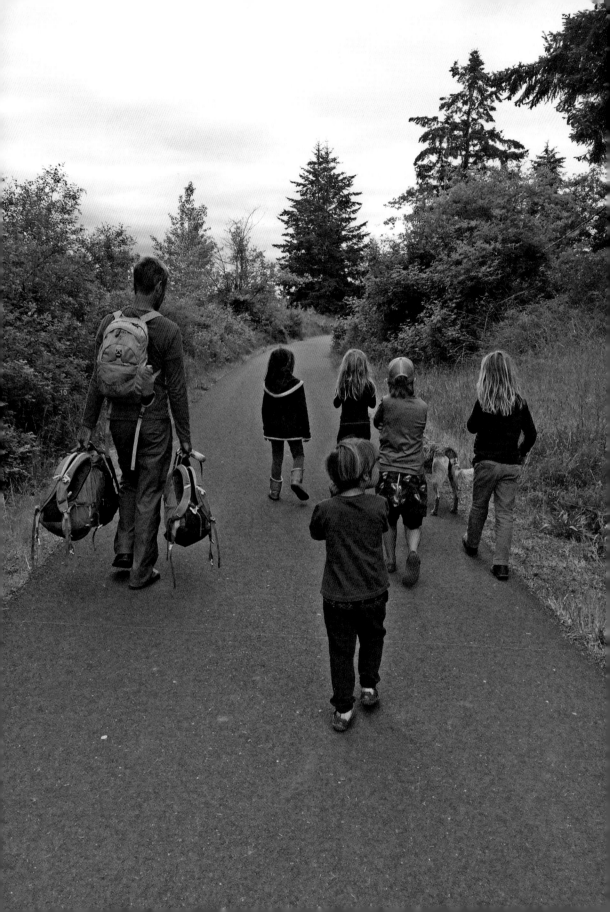

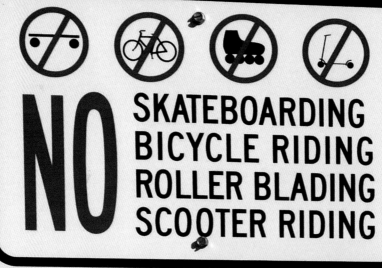

NO SKATEBOARDING BICYCLE RIDING ROLLER BLADING SCOOTER RIDING

SNP-103   PEACHTREE   1-800-241-4623   PBP1.com

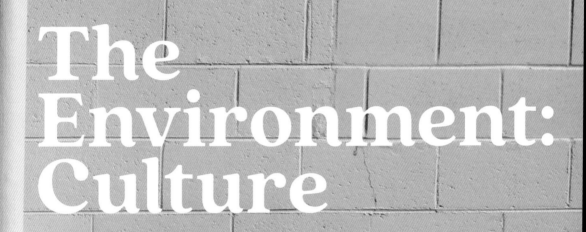

The Environment: Culture

Culture is an individual's set of attitudes, values, beliefs, and behaviors, as well as those shared by a group of people, communicated from one generation to the next.

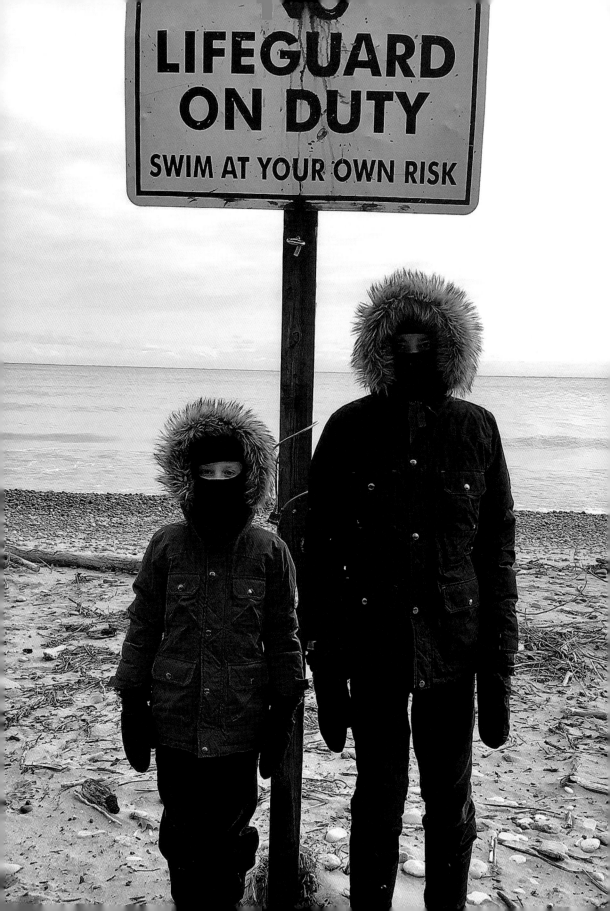

The Culture Container

chapter two

CULTURE HAS WALLS

It's easy to understand that a greenhouse is a container for a plant, a pair of shoes is a container for your feet, or a chair is a container for your body. We think of containers as having tangible sides and lids; we understand how physical barriers can keep us from moving. If your shoes are too tight and press your toes together, they stop your foot-parts moving around. Simple, once you think about it (more on footwear in chapter three). Understanding that CULTURE is *also* a container is more complicated, because even though culture directly impacts the physical shapes of things like buildings, furniture, and clothing, a lot of how a culture affects our movement is intangible. Its barriers are harder to identify.

A culture provides both the hardware and the software of our daily operating systems. This means it includes all the physical items that influence a group of people—the food, the silverware it might be eaten with, and tables it might be eaten upon; the calendars and signs upon the walls, as well as the walls themselves—but culture is not limited to these physical items. Culture also includes the attitudes, values, beliefs, and behaviors shared by a group of people. A culture can share the beliefs that it's unacceptable to chew with your mouth open, to talk with your mouth full (or to talk at all, as in "children should be seen and not heard"), or to put your elbows on the table. We each have our own personal culture, and we also belong to groups of people with whom we share beliefs and attitudes. We may have a family-of-origin culture, a community/location culture, a religious-/spiritual-community culture, an education culture, and more. Sometimes we examine our cultures and subcultures with awareness, and sometimes we participate and pass them on to our children without thinking about it much.

With the exception of NATURE, CULTURE is the largest of the environments we each operate within each day (see handy diagram next page). Culture is also the environment that contains all the other environments covered in this book.

While culture is an immense environment, it makes for the shortest chapter because I'll deal with the way culture influences various environments (e.g., movement at school and how we choose clothes that affect our movement) in each section of the book.

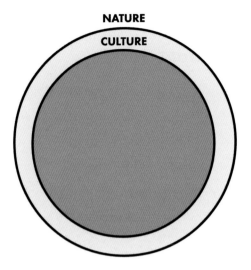

NATURE

CULTURE

But there's still plenty I need to say about culture here. I'm not a sociolo-gist; I'm a biomechanist. The aspects of culture I spend my time analyzing are those associated with movement. Inactivity, also known as sedentarism, is not only unprecedentedly widespread—it's also *increasing*. Not only are more people moving less, but the tiny amount of movement we have been doing is still decreasing. How is this possible? What is it about our society that makes *not* moving so easy? My quick answer is that it's due to our amazing ability to tinker and develop new technologies (from the first rudimentary wheels to fuel-guzzling machines like cars, planes, and internet servers), paired with our tendency to resist discomfort and conserve our energy. The result is a widespread culture that dissuades or blatantly prevents people from moving. Children born into this culture unconsciously adopt the practices, beliefs, and values of not moving. As adults continue to pass on sedentarism, each generation loses more movement than the one before.

NATURE AND "NATURE"

Nature from the broadest perspective is everything in the physical world (including physical laws), which means that culture is also part of nature. As I discussed on page 44, when we speak of nature, we are most often referring only to wild spaces, green and blue spaces, and areas that have trees, birds, bugs, rocks, and their unique microbiome. We use the term nature to mean all of the parts of the universe that don't include humans or the stuff humans make. Our current understanding of nature is really more like "nature" because it's so much smaller than what nature actually is.

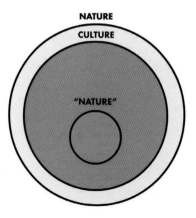

Our very narrow definition of nature is part of what keeps us from seeing that nature is more than green and wild stuff; nature includes guiding principles that our bodies, like all living things, must follow (we have to eat certain nutrients, drink fresh water, move, rest, etc.). Despite the way our culture views nature, our bodies are not something to take for a visit into "nature"; they're already part of the natural world.

The human elements of the world have become so all-encompassing that it makes it hard to see that we are still elements of nature. We are animals that, despite having the ability to organize a variety of societies, and create massive civilizations and impressive technologies, still have long-established biological needs. To meet those, we need nature (the green and wild spaces) to take up more space—in our lives and on the planet. We need our time in "nature" to take up more space in our lives.

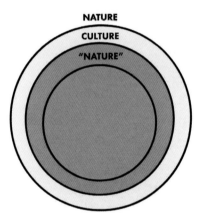

Even though humans have used up a large portion of nature in order to multiply themselves, it's important to remember that we still operate within the rules of the larger nature system.

To keep things easy I use the most conventional "wilderness/outdoor spaces/green and blue spaces" definition of nature in this book. I use this conventional definition because it is important to be clear how *little* time humans—especially small, developing humans—spend interacting with the non-human elements of the world. However, it's imperative that as we consider where our culture places humans in relation to nature, we keep this often-forgotten relationship in mind: we are a part of nature. Nature includes us.

MOVEMENT IS COUNTERCULTURE

I can't write a book about getting kids moving more without addressing the giant elephant in the room. This massive elephant is filling the room, blocking the windows and pinning shut the door to "more movement." Our elephant is this: **Movement is currently counterculture.** The way children move today has everything to do with the physical spaces and cultural practices we've collectively developed, as well as the values we've placed upon moving…and not moving. Kids moving around in a robust, dynamic way that develops and maintains their bodies are often thought of as dirty, noisy, and dangerous. Kids are told to sit still, stop climbing, don't run in here. Kids moving in a robust way do not fit in well with our collective and sometimes personal cultural values, even though we understand that "exercise is good." We've taken movement out of most areas of life and then approached kids' natural energy and need and capacity for movement by putting them into scheduled, structured, and limited movement sessions to use up their energy so that they *don't* run in the house, fidget in class, or stay active in other sedentary spaces we've created.

Any efforts to make changes that are counter to current culture can be met with resistance and frowning faces, and that's true of getting kids moving more. Most of the disapproval is reflexive because *any* change challenges the energy-conserving tendency within us all. But an even greater barrier is the fact that folks in this culture have moved so little that we don't fully grasp the elements, function, or importance of movement.

It's my work to clarify the phenomenon of movement—the history of it, the language used to describe and measure it, and the ways it operates as part of our anatomy. We all share responsibility to become aware of the way we shape access to movement in our personal and collective spaces. Our first exercise, when it comes to moving more, is to start noticing how much we discourage movement.

There are plenty of explicit rules about moving posted on tangible signs. No Running. No Jumping. No Climbing. Walking Not Permitted. Please Stay Off the Grass. These signs can be helpful—they're often safety-related and inform us of other people's expectations about how we should conduct ourselves in a given space.

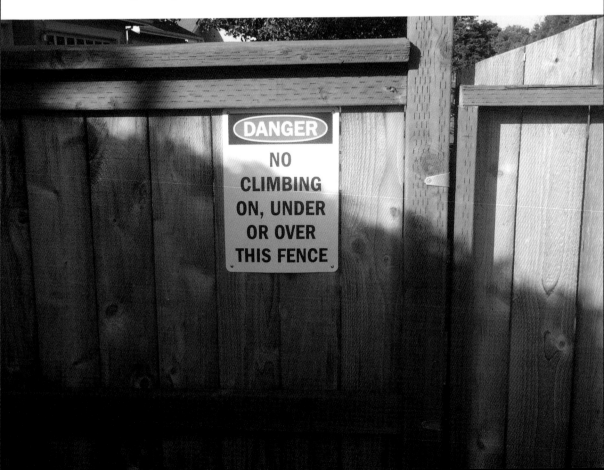

GIVE PERMISSION TO MOVE, EXPLICITLY

We're a very safety-minded, rule-abiding culture that tells kids multiple times a day that *their movement isn't tolerated* and, in many cases, is *breaking the rules*.

Activities like climbing and jumping can be risky, but in addition to building bodies, they build experience. Not being able to move robustly—with balance, skill, and judgment—can also put kids at risk. We love our kids so much (I get this!), but in our diligence to keep them from harm, we've forgotten to communicate where movement *is* permitted.

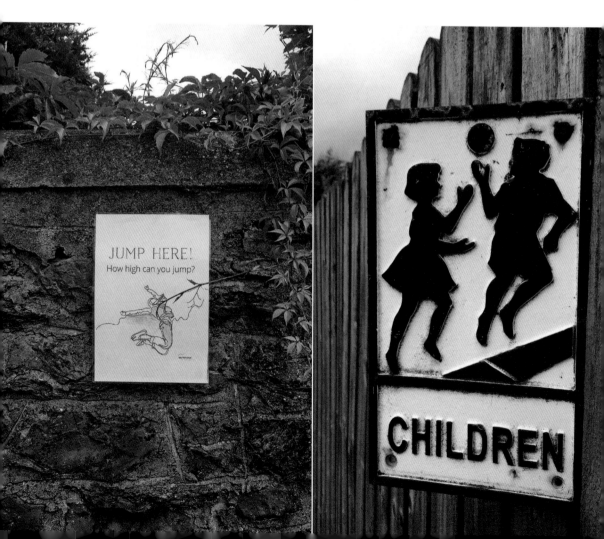

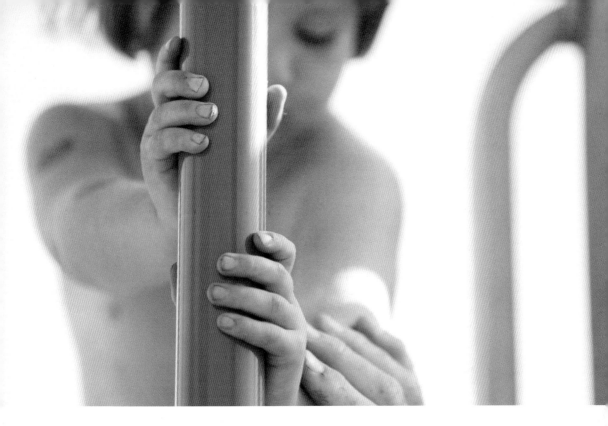

If we've agreed that information needs to be given in signs, then we must balance NO MOVEMENT HERE with a redirection. We need signs that communicate "Yeah, you can't do that over here, but it's perfectly fine to jump or roughhouse right over there."

Many signs have to do with safety, but many rules that we have about movement *don't* relate to safety. Rather they are more about the norms or daily operations of a sedentary culture. Why, for example, is everyone encouraged to take a seat most places? Is taking a seat different from quietly standing, squatting, or sitting on the floor? Is the noise from children jumping debilitating to those who hear it? Does another's fidgeting interfere with our daily life?

In the case of movement rules, we can ask, "Has this system been developed considering the needs of many people, including children? Is it possible to change our rules so that we can have a functioning society and not be disturbed by other people moving? When the only problem with someone moving in a space is *our perception that movement doesn't belong there*, is it possible to change our feelings about being bothered?"

It is in these spaces, where safety isn't an issue and sedentariness is a preference or habit, that we have the greatest opportunity to change the invisible barriers to movement. Why is it disruptive to stand or squat while waiting for an appointment? What is so awful about a kid jumping up and down in line, if they're not bumping into anyone?

GIVE PERMISSION TO MOVE, IMPLICITLY

There's another cultural aspect of human movement that is often unexplored. As adults in a society, we continuously teach, via modeling, what kids need to learn in order to be a successful adult. When the adults around them aren't moving frequently, what does this communicate to children? If adult society requires a tremendous amount of stillness, and childhood is when young humans prepare their bodies and minds to be successful in the adult world, then it's no wonder children are barely moving. If we want children to move more, they need to see movement being done more often. One of the easiest ways to get kids to move more and to value movement more is to give them unspoken permission to do so simply by moving more yourself.

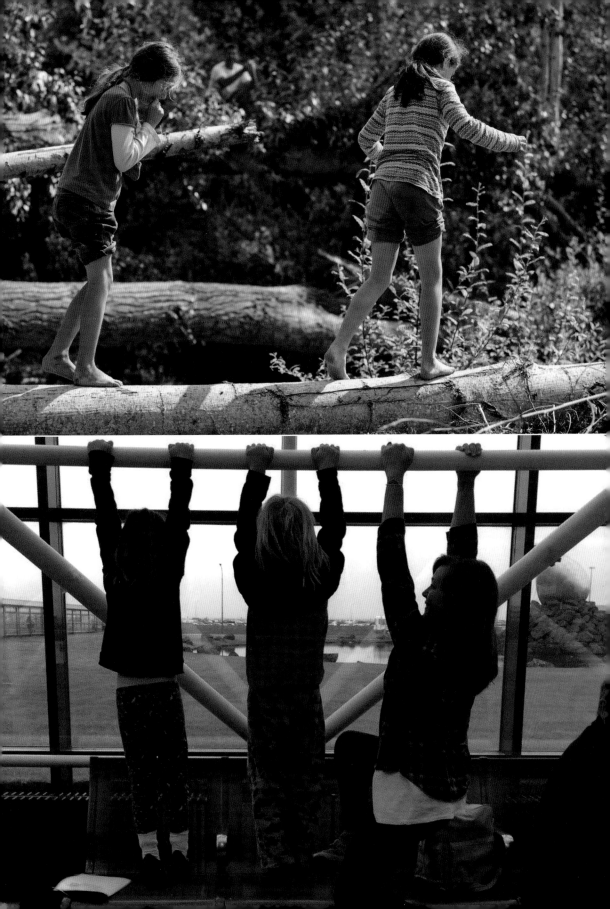

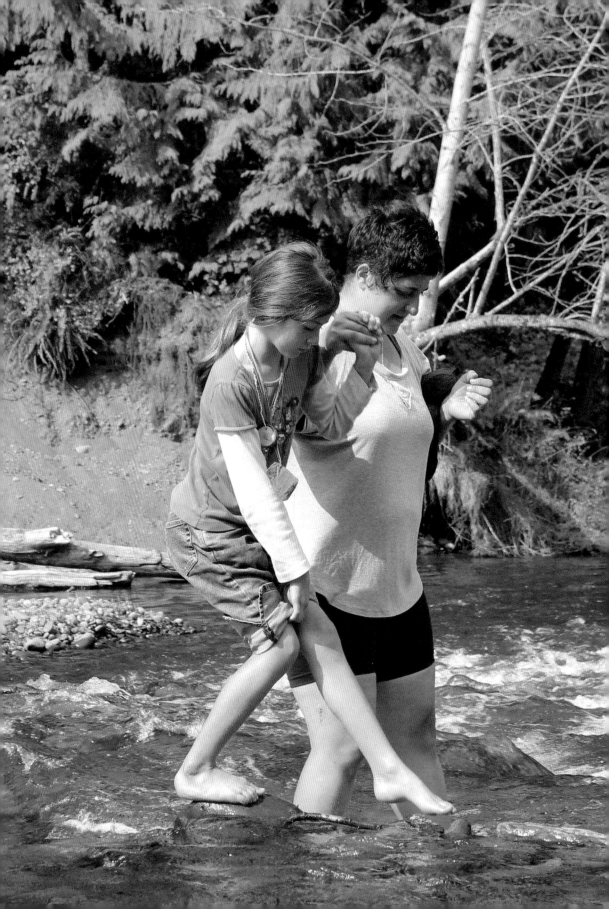

WHAT DOES A DYNAMIC CULTURE LOOK LIKE?

To see what a sedentary culture looks like, just look around. Not only at how the people inside of it are moving, but the structures they're moving within. What is it in our surrounding environment that prevents movement or encourages a lack of it? Anything that allows us to get away with not moving is part of a sedentary culture. The push of the button, tapping of the keys, and swipe of a thumb have become the acceptable stand-in for all the movements that used to be necessary for getting whatever you needed.

In a dynamic culture where there are more people moving, the environment will look different—not only because of the amount of nature present, but in the built environment as well. A dynamic culture has:

- homes with rules and spaces that let their inhabitants be dynamic
- schooling that encourages movement beyond a physical education session
- towns and cities with paths or streets that can be walked and rolled along safely, and can be used for everyday active transport as well as recreation
- plenty of green and wild spaces, accessible to all
- a "movement quotient" rating for new technologies, and a process in families, schools, and governments for choosing which technologies to adopt and which to leave behind

As we work toward a culture that sees and prioritizes movement over sedentarism, you won't only see more kids "get exercise"; their movement opportunities will be abundant throughout the day and permeate the structures of previously sedentary spaces.

SMALL STEPS MAKE BIG CHANGES

Movement and moving more are very personal. In each chapter you'll find both built environment and movement habits to play with, ranging from small cultural elements (like a dynamic wardrobe) to large ones (like advocating for more recess time). Don't be overwhelmed by the many ways you can move more; just identify and start with the opportunities that resonate the most with you, your family, and your situation. Overhauling a culture, specifically the larger framework of beliefs and attitudes that aren't tethered to a particular place or event, is big work. It's important work, but huge challenges such as changing the culture of a school district or the perceptions of what your community perceives as acceptable clothing for kids aren't always the easiest place to begin.

Fortunately, each environment is full of small changes you can make in your own personal and family culture that restore a child's freedom to move. **You don't need a giant shift in the culture to get kids moving more**; by changing how you and your family move, *you* change the movement culture—and by modeling it, you make it easier for others to move and change their culture as well.

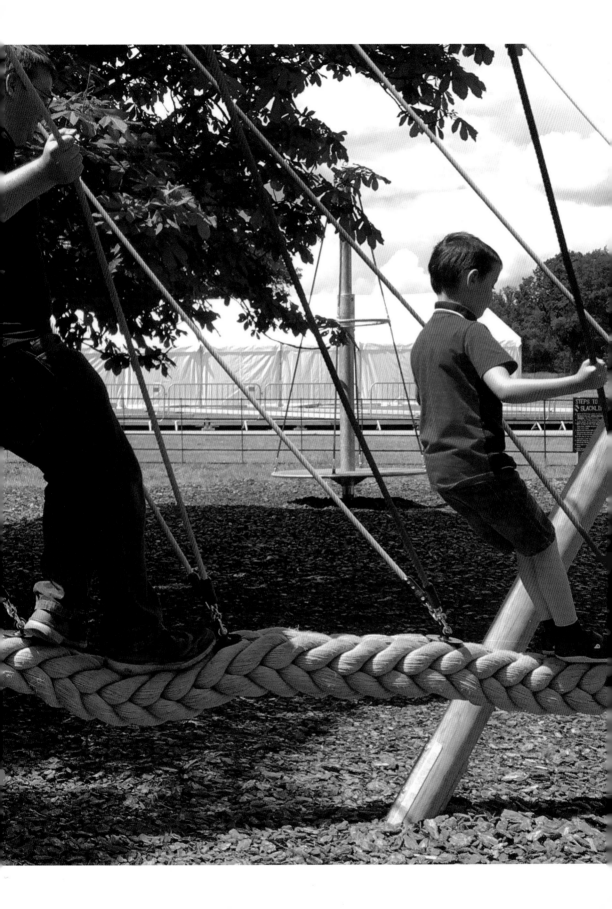

STEPS TO
SLACKLINE

MOVEMENT BIAS CHECK-IN: CULTURE

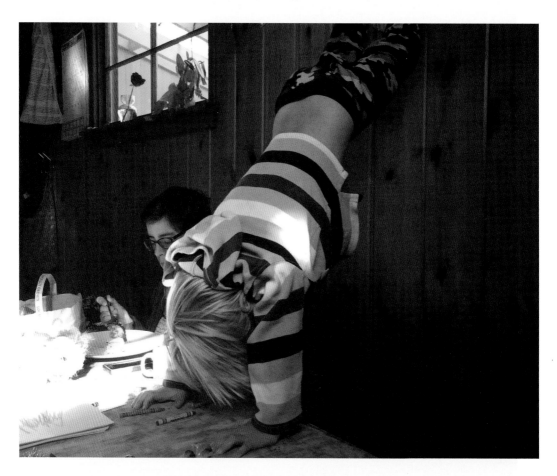

I'm not only a movement educator; I'm also a parent. I know what it's like to feel uncomfortable when my children's movement disrupts a sedentary space. It is so much easier to force the movement out of our kids than to put the movement back into our culture.

In each of the environment sections ahead, I'll pose questions that will help you figure out your attitudes, values, and beliefs around movement in various arenas of life.

While we have enough in common to be able to say "our culture," we also have our own unique set of subcultures, including our personal one, that affects our individual as well as collective behavior. So as people creating and taking care of children's environments, we can check in with ourselves to see where we might be able to permit more movement.

Here's your first set of questions, to work on personally or as a family, a school, or any other place children pass through.

In the spaces you're in charge of facilitating,

- **What are any written or explicit rules about movement? What are the reasons for each rule?**
- **How do/would you feel when kids sit on the floor or climb on chairs rather than sitting on them? What does it mean to you when they do?**
- **Do you have any signs giving permission to move or indicating where movement is okay?**
- **In what percentage of your space is movement possible? Are you open to changing your space in some way to increase that percentage?**
- **Do you feel movement is beneficial to children? How is it beneficial? Which parts of their lives or bodies benefit from movement? Which types of movement? What frequency of movement do they require?**
- **Where do you think children should be moving? What spaces are allotted to these types of movement? How do you facilitate the needs you believe they have?**

STUDY SESSION: WHY I SIT

Many people are aware kids are becoming more sedentary, and many are working on interventions. Some emerging ideas include reducing screen time, using movement trackers so wearers can objectively see their amount of movement, and setting movement goals. However, research into the cultural aspects of sedentarism shows that the top reasons children are inactive are "I sit because of the norm/I sit because I have to," "I sit because I can work/play better that way," and "I sit because there is nobody to play with." So researchers

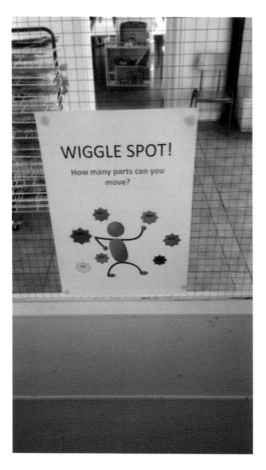

point out that all these "must sit" reasons might contribute greatly to sedentary behavior. They suggest that instead of focusing on setting activity goals, it might be more effective for adults to address any cultural contributions by tolerating or even encouraging more physical activity during lessons, homework time, or screen time in both home and school environments.

Hidding, L., T.M. Altenburg, E. van Ekris, and M.J.M. Chinapaw. "Why Do Children Engage in Sedentary Behavior? Child- and Parent-Perceived Determinants." *International Journal of Environmental Research and Public Health*, June 22, 2017.

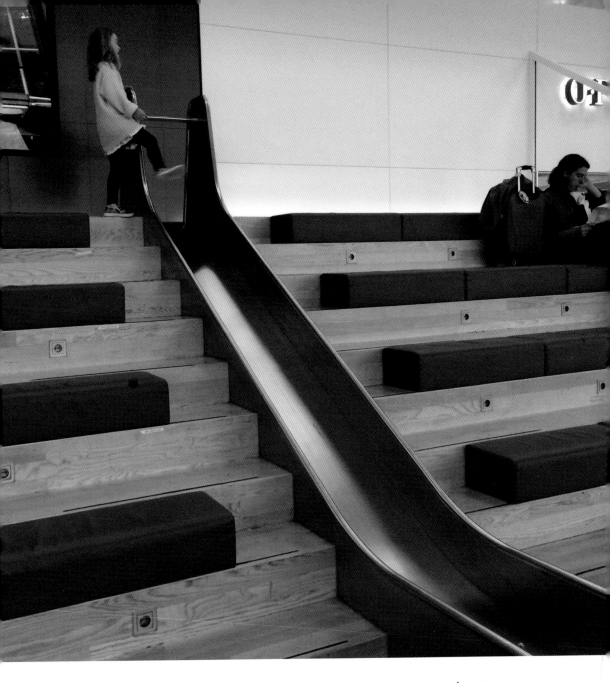

Travel requires a lot of sitting. Sitting to get to the airport, sitting at the airport, sitting on the plane. Some airports have toddler play areas where kids can freely do their thing away from others, but in the Amsterdam airport, movement opportunities like this slide have been built in the waiting areas. Movement isn't relegated to one small room in an otherwise huge environment; a little movement is made possible within all waiting areas. Movement and play are normalized, and P.S. I went down this slide a couple times myself.

SHOW AND TELL

Mindset has been the biggest thing that has had to shift for me in order to create a movement-friendly environment for my kids (and myself). I realized that "Don't climb on that," "Sit still," and "Sit down" had become automatic responses to my children's behavior.

Recently I was filling some pots up with compost. My children (ages six and two) started playing with a bag of compost that was lying on the ground. They took a run up, jumped on it, and then jumped off, pretending it was a gymnastics springboard. The first thought that went through my mind was to tell them, "Stop it, you are supposed to be filling pots," but I caught that thought...My kids were being creative, working together as a team, and getting some great movement-nutrients, so I encouraged them. Later they came and helped me fill up the pots too (adding another dimension of movement).

My kids are really good at creating their own movement opportunities, but I used to discourage it for fear of it being unsafe, too noisy, or just not the done thing. I think culture was a big hindrance for me.

—Hannah Hall

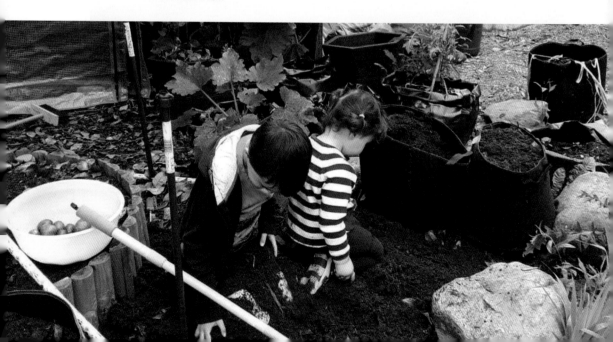

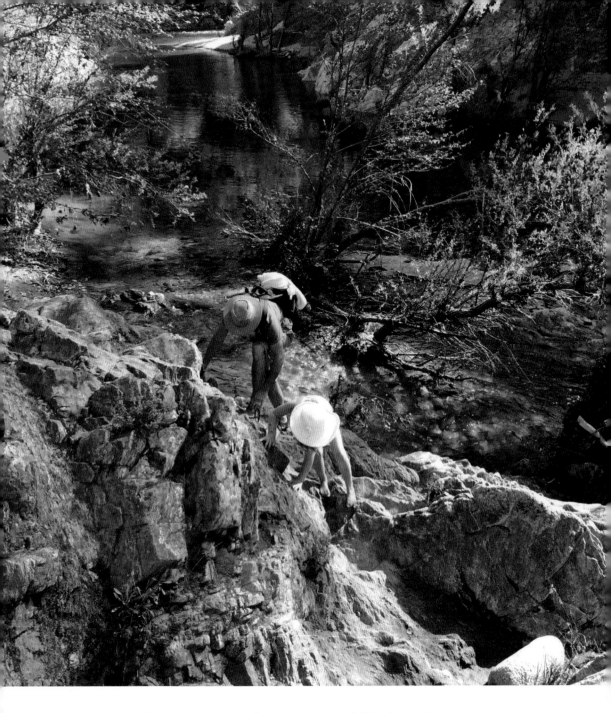

There's a cyclical aspect to my family's parent-child relationship to
moving. Having grown up sedentary, my husband and I had to work
to create an environment where abundant movement is allowed. But
as we watch and follow our kids as they move intuitively through
that environment, we're constantly inspired to move more ourselves.
Co-learning for the win!

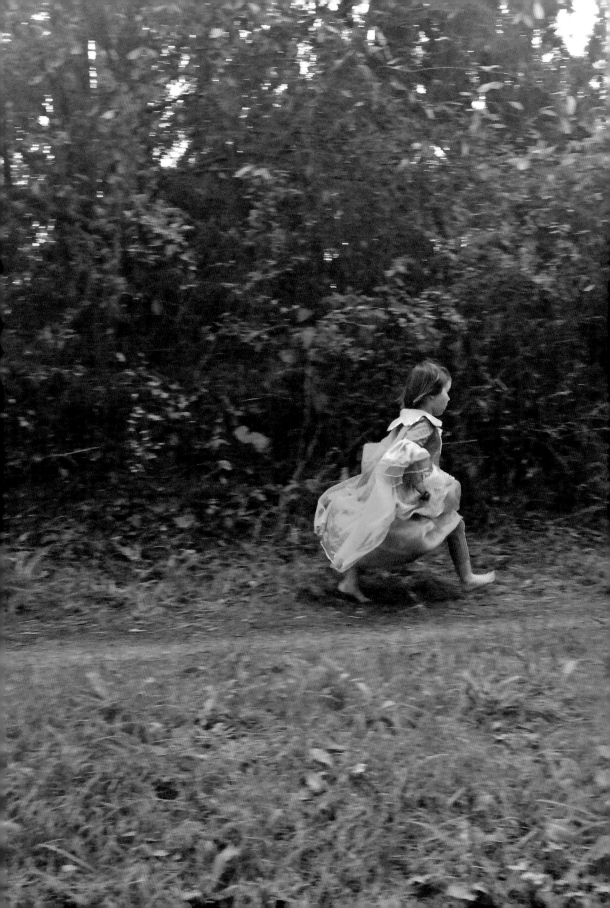

The Environment: Apparel

Apparel is what we wear—clothing (including shoes, hats, backpacks, etc.) that covers our body to keep it warm or protected from environmental hazards (thorns, sun, cold, etc.), as well as to express our individual or cultural style.

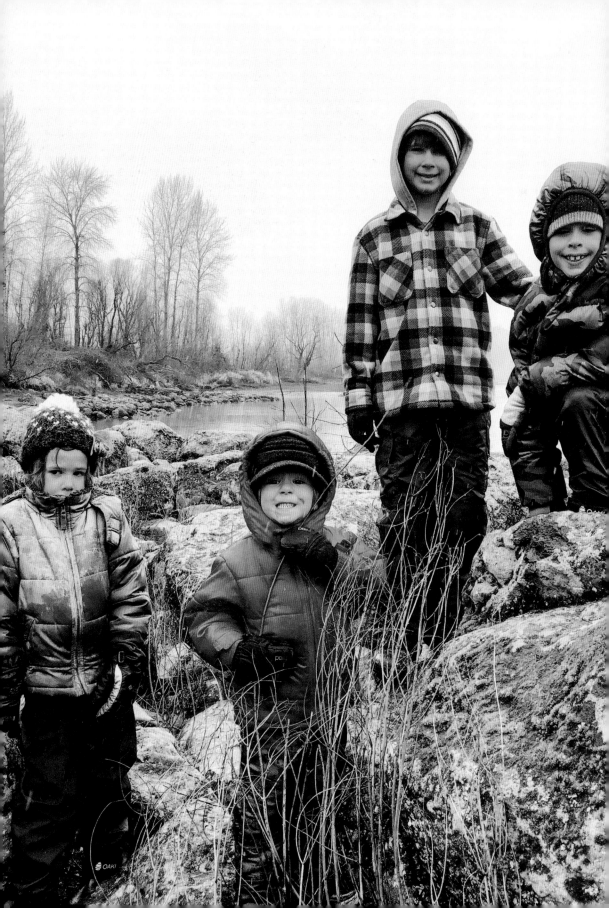

The Clothing Container

chapter three

I'm betting that you're wearing clothes as you read this.

Did I win?

Second to culture, we likely spend more time *within* our clothing than we do inside any other single environment. We tell our children to go get some clothes *on*, but what we're really having them do is get *into* their clothing. The shoes and pants they wear wrap *around* their toes, ankles, knees, and hips; belts, shirts, and jackets *contain* their abdomens, shoulders, and arms. Kids are *inside* their clothes, so the way their clothing stretches and bends becomes the way a child can stretch or bend. To think of it another way: a child's outfit is a container for their movement.

I first tuned in to the effects of kid clothing when I took my two-year-old to a playground we knew well. As we made the regular laps around familiar equipment, I watched him try to mount his favorite sandbox rocking horse while wearing a pair of jeans for the first time, just handed down from his cousin. He strained to lift his leg up and over the horse once, then twice, to no avail. I finally realized that his jeans were resisting this familiar motion and keeping his legs together! I also saw him, without any fuss, give up on trying to make the necessary straddling movement to get on the horse and instead walk to another area of the park.

If he hadn't been to the playground before and ridden this horse in more flexible pants, and if I hadn't been paying attention to him trying and failing to get on the horse, it would have been easy to chalk up his passing on this experience as his personal preference or lack of ability rather than what it was: his new clothes were preventing him from moving. It only took the quiet resistance of his pants to keep him from moving in a particular way—a way he loved to move.

There are many ways to evaluate clothing. There's how it looks, how much it costs, how well it will wear, and how it was made. But there is also how it moves. Natural kid movement is not only constant—it's varied, too. Running, jumping, climbing, swinging, balancing, bending, hopping, twisting, squatting, crawling, digging, carrying, lifting, exploring. When you need to use a variety of body shapes each day, your clothing has to adjust to make these movements possible.

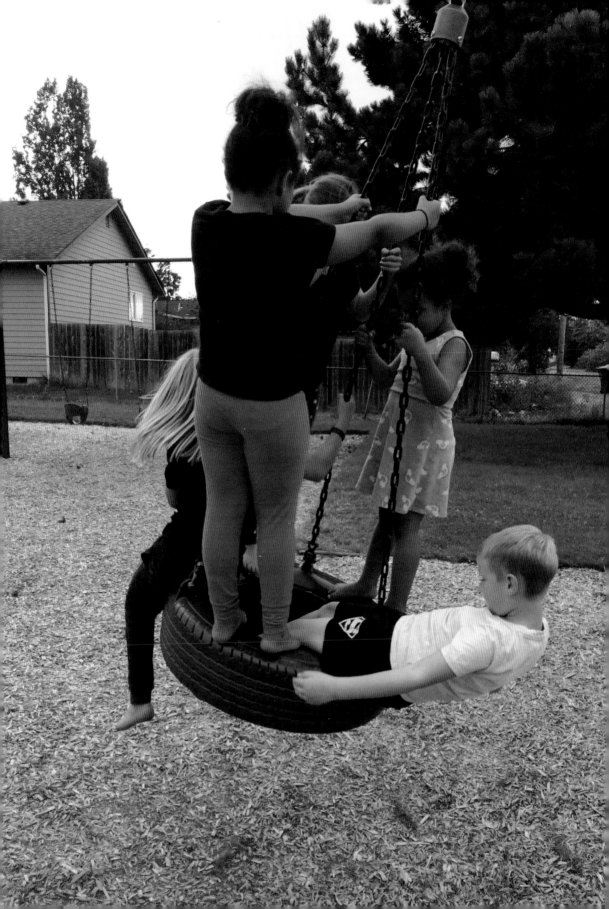

MOVEMENT BIAS CHECK-IN: APPAREL

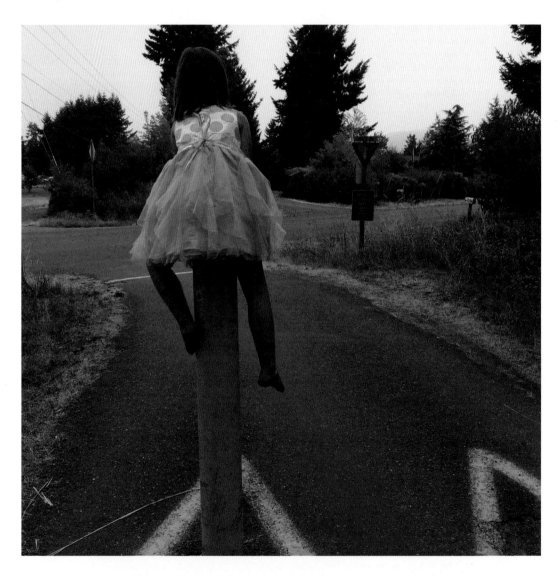

I grew up having "nice clothes" and "play clothes," and I also grew up watching *The Sound of Music*, where old curtains will forever be part of the clothing necessary for climbing trees.

I'm not sure if anyone ever talked about it with me directly or whether I just knew that nice clothes were for times when it was expected we looked neat—very sedentary times (church, holiday gatherings, school concerts). I also knew that nice clothes should stay neat and intact, and how could I keep them that way and do anything other than sit inside?

Let's check in with our movement biases around clothes.

- **Did you grow up with explicit or implicit rules around clothing and keeping it clean or nice? What were the consequences for breaking those rules?**

- **What are your family's current explicit or implicit rules to dirtying or wearing out clothing? How did those rules come to be? What are the feelings you have when your kids break those rules?**

- **What do dirty/damaged clothes communicate to you? To others? Can you think of anyone, a relative or story character, who has an iconic costume that is torn or dirt-laden that you find pleasing? (For me, this is Indiana Jones.) What does this character's dirty/damaged clothing communicate to you?**

- **Do you/your family currently distinguish between school and play clothes? Special-occasion clothes? What is the ratio of these outfits?**

- **Do you have moving and non-moving clothing? What movements do you do in your moving clothes and in which spaces? How dirty (as in actual dirt vs. sweat) do your moving clothes get?**

IF THEY'RE NOT "PLAY CLOTHES," WHAT ARE THEY?

Adults have "movement" clothes, categories of outfits they get into when it's time for exercise. Even if you don't call them your workout or play clothes, we acknowledge the need for more dynamic outfits by putting them on when it's time for us to get moving. Because we move so little throughout the day, dynamic clothing is the exception, not the rule. This is why we can see and even label "exercise clothes" but we don't consciously view (and we certainly don't label) the outfits that make up our weekly wardrobe as our "sedentary clothes." Still, the bulk of what many of us choose to wear each day is designed for the stationary sitting hours that fill our day.

There are many symptoms of a sedentary culture that keep our sedentary ways growing. The folks who design environments—like clothing—for children likely grew up in a sedentary culture and don't have a robust movement perspective themselves. The adults selecting clothes might not think of the ways clothing allows or prevents movement, and can easily opt for the culture's conventional clothing. "Sedentary clothing," for a sedentary culture, is simply "clothing," and culturally appropriate clothing makes up most of a child's wardrobe, hindering their movement—not even on purpose.

The great news is that sedentary cultures aren't grown willfully (I don't think folks are *trying* to convince everyone, let alone their children, to move less), but rather they exist because we haven't yet identified all the ways in which we don't or can't move, or how our environment prevents us from moving. Once you identify the way clothing influences movement, you will recognize it, and that awareness gives you the option to change things up for more movement, in yourselves and in kids.

THE IMPACT OF CLOTHES THAT FIT *AND FIT IN*

Most clothing is designed for a person standing squarely with feet slightly apart and arms at the sides. Designers make sure uniform and athletic gear can support performance or offer protection without hindering the necessary motion, but very little attention has been paid to children's clothing and how it might help or hinder activity levels.

Compounding the issue is the fact that kids come in different shapes and sizes. As more and more children wrestle with obesity issues, clothing can further hinder movement because shirts and pants are often designed with the assumption that if you have a larger waist, you also have longer arms and legs.

Beyond some small-group research I've been able to find (see this chapter's reference section) there's been little attention paid to the fact that larger-waisted pre-teens and teenagers who want to move more might not have acccess to clothing that fits well and also meets the very important need to also look good or at least like they fit in. If we have to put on an adult size T-shirt to go over our waist, the fact that it's too long for our body binds our legs together. Maybe adult-size sweatpants are comfortable around the waist, but the extra fabric at the ankles is cumbersome and can be a drag—both literally and figuratively. My point is, clothing is often a statement of who we are, and

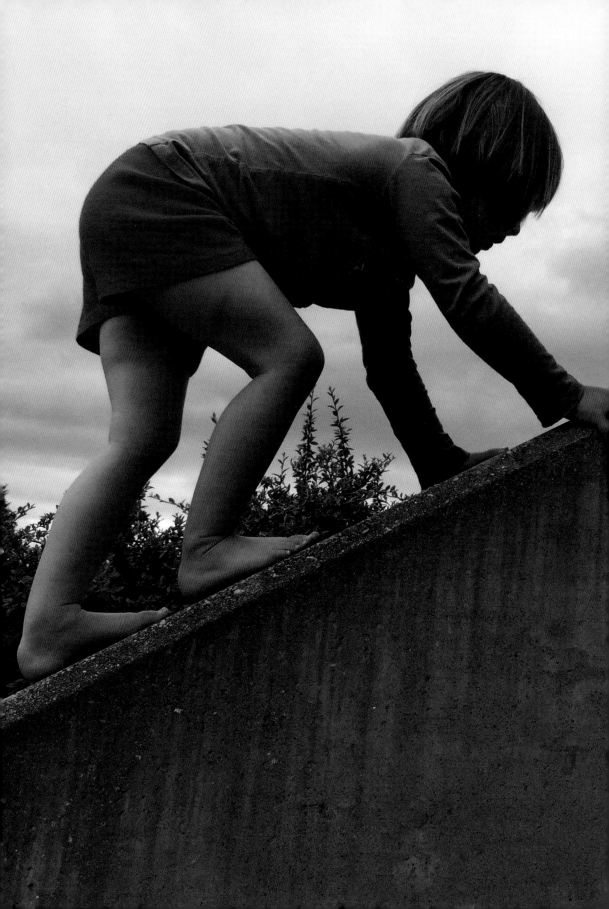

if there are no clothes that allow a kid with a bigger waist to be active and stylish, then how can we expect them to feel good about moving?

If you think this could be an issue for your child, talk to them about it. You can often find a tailor who can make adjustments to a few outfits (start with any required PE outfits) so their exercise clothes fit well and look good. Find that relative who's got wicked sewing skills and spend some time with your teen designing an all-day dynamic outfit or two, or be our hero and start a dynamic kids' clothing company with stylish options at a variety of waist sizes.

SEDENTARY SHOES

Shoes, at the most basic level, are clothing for the feet. Clothing has to be flexible so the body can move; shoes have to be flexible so feet can move.

Feet are dynamic by nature and need movement to stay healthy. Each foot has thirty-three joints and each of these has to move. Some foot joints can only change position a little. Stepping on bumpy terrain, rocks, and other nature-bits keeps them moving. Other joints in the feet, like those in the toes and the ankles, are much more mobile and are kept dynamic via activities like walking over up-and-down terrain, squatting, sitting on the ground, and climbing.

Shoes offer a layer of protection for the feet, but when it comes to moving well, we need to understand the difference between providing our feet with a barrier from sharp objects and wearing shoes so stiff that the bulk of our foot parts can't articulate. It's likely that your own closet is full of shoes that don't let your feet move, so this set of shoe tests can be done as a family.

HOW FLEXIBLE IS THE SHOE?

In order for the joints and muscles in your feet to move, they have to be able to bend around the shape of whatever you're walking over (see page 100 for more on how walking surfaces move us). Try bending the front of the shoe towards the back of the shoe. Look for shoes that bend fairly easily in this direction.

What about its lengthwise flexibility? Try twisting the heel and toe of the shoe in opposite directions. Look for shoes that are malleable enough to resemble the shape of a cinnamon twist.

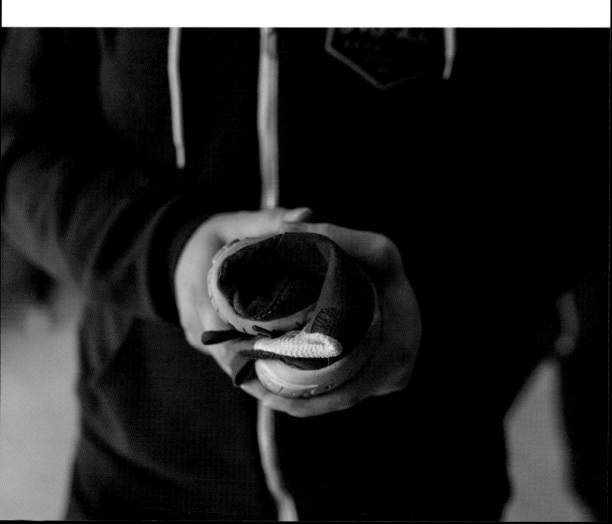

IS THERE SPACE FOR DYNAMIC TOES?

Toe movements include lifting, curling, and spreading. When you're walking, there's not a ton of curling and spreading needed, but toe spreading is always helpful for balance and stability. You and your child can stand up and gently curl your toes, as if your shoes were a little too short. Notice how that decreases the width of the front of your foot. Then, try to spread your toes away from each other, noticing how that widens the front of your foot.

Next, stand on a piece of paper. Spread your toes and trace your feet, then set your shoes over the top of your drawing to see if your feet are wider than your shoes. In order for your toes to be able to move when you're out moving the rest of your body, select shoes that don't force your toes together like a stiff-legged pair of jeans.

HOW HIGH ARE THE HEELS?

Conventional shoes, for whatever reason, include heels. And I don't only mean the heels on kid-sized dress shoes, but the heels you'll find on school shoes and soccer shoes, summer sandals, toddler shoes, and even "healthy shoes for kids." If you look at the kid shoes around you, you'll probably find that, like adult shoes, there's a heel on almost every pair.

A heeled shoe creates a slight downhill position of the ankle, prevents the full range of motion of the ankle, and also moves the center of pressure to the front of the foot. Such shoes therefore change the body's weight distribution and its ability to balance and stabilize.

The height of the heel might not seem like much (maybe about an inch). But kids have short feet, and that magnifies the effect of even a heel of seemingly inconsequential height.

This means that, in the case of these shoes (a man's size 11 and a child's size 1), the angle between the standing surface and the foot is much greater in the child than in the adult. Children's shoes are not *mini* versions of adult fashion; they're *maxi* versions.

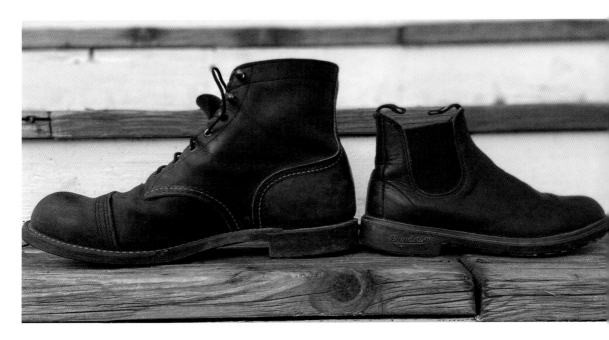

Shoes worn for medical issues, playing sports, dancing, or the occasional dress-up time are not a huge problem. It's what we wear *most* of the time that matters. Focus on choosing more dynamic shoes that are worn for the greatest amount of time.

TAKE THE CHALLENGING SURFACE CHALLENGE

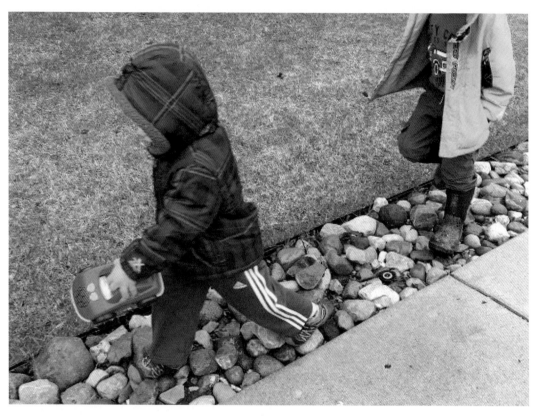

Flexible shoes are made to allow the ground to move all the joints in your feet more, but they can only do that when what you walk on is lumpy. Flat-and-level ground in flexible shoes is still just flat and level. Seek out texture on your walks as you'd seek out items in a scavenger hunt. Can you find rocky pathways to walk over, with lumps and bumps that get the feet and ankles moving more? Kids are like super-computers with their ability to look for and retain patterns. Show them what texture looks like and encourage them to take the path more cobbled.

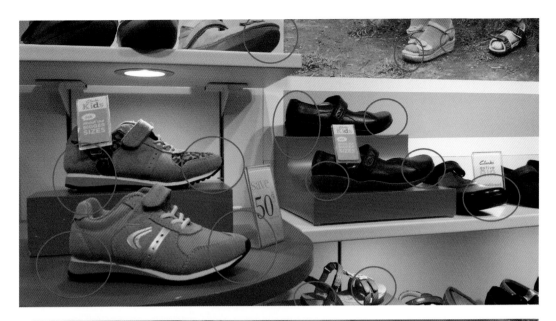

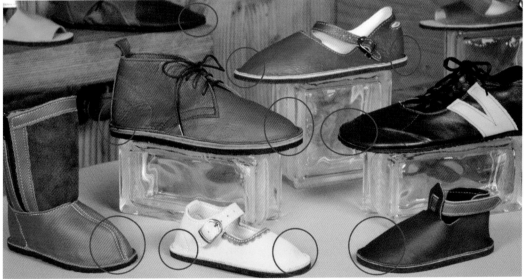

Once you start really looking at footwear's geometry, you'll see how shoes can look very different from the feet they're meant to fit! I've circled all the elevated heels and toe-boxes in the top picture so you can better evaluate the shoes in your own closet.

Minimal footwear offers the same foot protection while minimally altering the shape and motion of the wearer's foot. I've circled the heels and toes in the lower picture (these are Softstar brand) so you can see what "zero-rise" heels and level toe-boxes look like.

HOW WELL DO THE SHOES STAY ON?

A well-connected shoe is essential for an emerging mover. Slip-on shoes are also slip-*off* shoes unless your toes constantly grip to keep them on. Adding toe-gripping or shuffling patterns to walking can make walking difficult or uncomfortable. Shoes that easily slip off can also make a game of tag or a climbing session dangerous, if not downright impossible. Activities such as these can be labeled unsafe, but it's often the gear that sets kids up for potential injury.

HOW HEAVY (AND HOW HIGH) IS THE SHOE?

I've attended many nature classes for kids, and inevitably there are children who show up wearing boots that fit the length of their feet but are much too tall and/or heavy for easy movement. By passing over the ankles and preventing them from moving, tall boots can act a bit like a cast on a broken bone. Instead of being able to make fine ankle adjustments based on any lumps and bumps they encounter, kids with boot-casted ankles often end up lurching as they negotiate the terrain.

Heavy shoes can have a similar gait-altering effect. Imagine if someone tied light weights to your feet. Legs act as long levers, so adding even a light weight at the end of them creates excessive lurching or swinging motions. Even if kids can do the extra work to stabilize excessive motions caused by shoes, they might not want to walk far or long because it's so fatiguing.

Everyone's level of physical ability is different, and we can encourage each child to move as well as *they* can by making sure their movement environment, including shoes, doesn't create or worsen any issues. Look for light shoes, and low boots that flex easily at the ankle so they don't act like a cast and keep the ankle in one place.

WHAT TRACTION DOES THE SHOE OFFER?

It's *fun* to move well. Climbing is a joy, and a game of tag and other balance games—how far can you walk along this wobbly log? How long can you stand on it?—are an exciting way to interact with other children and the surrounding nature.

One of the reasons humans are such good climbers is that the skin on our hands and feet provides really good traction. When you add materials like plastic and rubber on top of that skin, make sure that these don't hinder climbing and balancing movements or make them more hazardous by removing our natural traction.

There's no perfect material or tread for a shoe; what you need depends on what you're doing, where you're doing it (are you on cement? metal? mud?), and how wet or otherwise slippery the surfaces you're traversing are. You can encourage your kids to pay attention to how their footwear feels as it moves over the ground. Are their running shoes fine on cement but too slick in the woods? Do their sandals grip the wet rocks well?

My kids did not wear shoes before they could walk. They had booties or socks for warmth when needed, but they also had lots of barefoot time. I thought of their hands and feet as the sensory organs they are, and wanted them to be able to learn the world by "looking" at things by pressing their feet against our bodies or other things inside and outside our home.

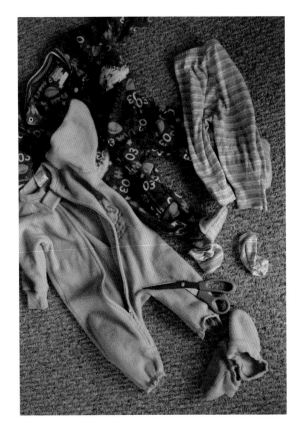

I also put them in feety (or is it footie?) pajamas, because that's what you do. *You put kids in feety pajamas.* Once they were crawling and starting to stand, I noticed that the pajama feet were a hindrance. With his hands grasping the coffee table, my son kept trying to pull up while pushing off with his feet. Only his feet kept sliding. Why? Because the slippery pajama feet provided no traction against our slippery floors. He was ready to stand, and his body parts were trying to join in, but the environment I had placed him in was making it so he couldn't get up.

I watched him for a good fifteen minutes, wondering what to do, before I realized what to do: cut the feet off his pajamas. So I did, and up he went, and the moral of the story is that sometimes something that takes care of one need (like feety pajamas giving warmth, or shoes giving protection) creates an issue elsewhere. We therefore need to think critically to figure out when a "solution" harms as much or more than it helps. Also, if anyone knows a crafty way to upcycle a pile of pajama feet, do let me know.

VITAMIN BAREFOOT

Foot coverings are necessary in many of the areas we need to move through. But there are some foot parts that cannot fully do their job if they're always inside shoes, even the most minimal shoes. For kids to move all of the parts of their body, and for their feet to develop the strength and shape that will serve them well in future, they need to spend time with their feet bare and moving in complex, challenging ways.

Watching a young child learn new ways to move is fascinating. The way a baby moves each finger in a slow, deliberate manner when trying to pick up an object or turn a knob shows how intensely children concentrate on learning how to move and how to manipulate their environment through movement.

Now imagine putting mittens on that infant or toddler as they learn to grasp, pick up a pea to eat, recognize the difference between hot, cold, textured, and smooth, turn a doorknob, hold a crayon, or write their name.

We wouldn't put mittens on baby hands trying to figure out how to grasp the world, and yet we don't think twice about covering their nerve-dense feet with rubber and cotton as they learn their very first movements. Trying to protect them from potential injury is understandable, but the way we have come to use kid footwear is like putting headphones on a baby right when they're trying to learn what the world around them sounds like.

Our culture tends to be hand-dominant. Perhaps because our feet were covered and contained from an early age, and because we don't use our feet (or other body parts) that much, the idea that the anatomy of our hands

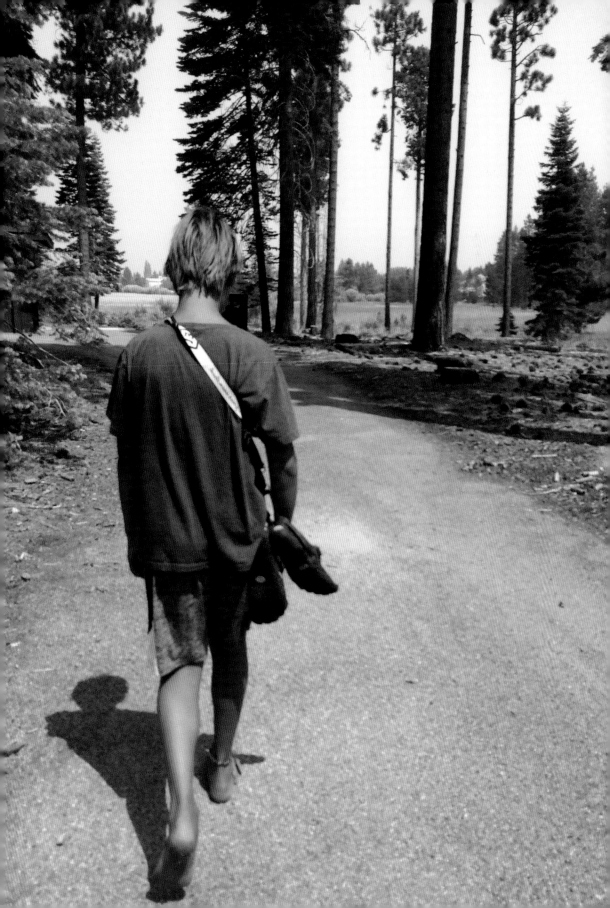

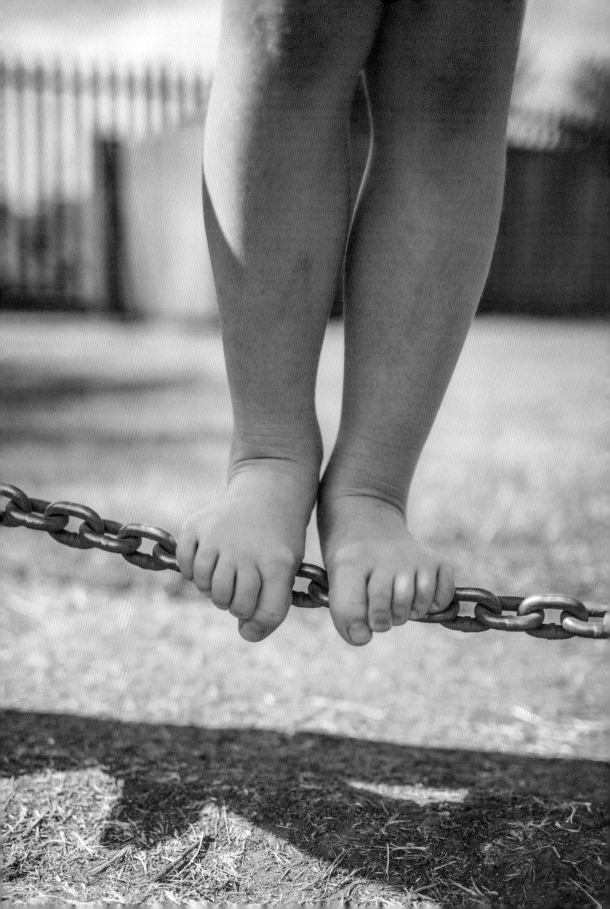

matches the anatomy of our feet sounds almost silly. But our toes and feet need to explore and send data to our brain in the same way our hands do, and the rest of our body needs to receive this information from the feet so it can organize the movements of walking and balancing. Sensory nerves are important to how our brains function.

Certainly it's not safe for youngsters to be barefoot in every space, but there are environments where it is possible, and one of those is likely your own home. Start there, and explore locally to look for natural spaces that can accommodate regular shoe-free movement time—these will generally be free of garbage and animal poop. Push for city park clean-ups or organize your own to help create safe barefoot places for more people.

SHOPPING FOR MINIMAL SHOES

Conventional shoes, by definition, have many customers, so they're mass-produced and available at much lower cost than more dynamic shoes (also known as "minimal shoes"), which are often made by smaller companies. This is a gentle way of explaining why minimal footwear is often more expensive.

Too-small shoes keep kids' feet and walking motions from developing well, which is why guidelines recommend their shoes should be at least half an inch (1.2 cm) longer than their foot. Children's feet are constantly growing, and a well-fitting shoe can quickly become too small. (And, P.S., buying shoes a full size larger than kids need is not recommended, as too-big shoes also make walking and balance a challenge.) Kids' rapid growth makes a well-fitting shoe a constantly moving target, and most kids will likely need at least two or three pairs of shoes per year, which quickly adds up.

I've been guiding families on minimal footwear for almost a decade, and they've been sharing their own tips and feedback with me, so here is a general approach we've figured out to reduce cost. You can find more specific shoe suggestions on my website by searching "minimal shoes."

Buy a pair of water (swim/pool) shoes at the beginning of the school year, and again mid-year. Water or pool shoes are usually pretty cheap (typically less than twenty bucks) and you can get at least two pairs throughout the year, accommodating foot growth without breaking the bank. The rubber sole of pool shoes means they're fine for walking on wet ground (although not great for puddle stomping), and paired with some wool socks, my kids are happy in them even in chilly (40°F) weather as long as it's not raining. These are the most affordable and available minimal shoes I've found for children.

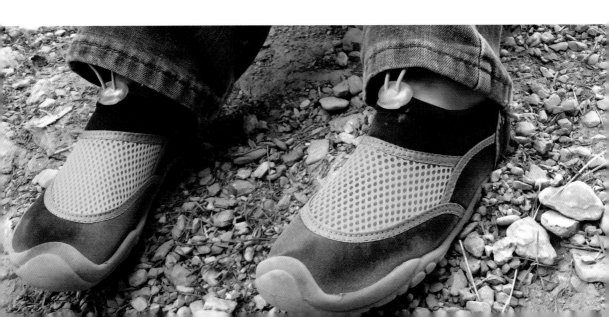

Don't buy "back to school" shoes in September. Often the early part of the school year has milder weather, so your kids can keep wearing their "summer" or fair-weather footwear a bit longer. If you're investing in a pair of well-made minimal shoes, order slightly later in the season, as late as November if you can get away with it, so your kids' "back to school/winter" pair of shoes covers more of the time when summer shoes just won't cut it. With any luck, by the time they need new shoes, water shoes will work just fine again.

The best time to try on shoes for fit is at the end of the day after kids have been up and moving around for a few hours. Feet can change size throughout the day, depending on use. Feet will be smaller in the early morning (after lying down for a long time) or after just sitting in school all day. For the best fit, try on shoes after a day of being upright and active.

Give them style autonomy. While our seven- and nine-year-old know our family looks for shoes that have certain features (flat, flexible, wide toe-box, etc.), part of letting them learn about their bodies and accommodating their need for self-expression is letting them look through styles they like and evaluating for themselves whether they pass the movement tests. Before shopping, have your child step on a piece of paper, spread their toes away from each other, and trace their foot. Having the tracing ready in the store lets children quickly measure shoes against the drawing instead of repeatedly coming to you to ask if each pair is okay. In this way, the process becomes less about these features being *my* rule and more a way of simply checking for themselves whether the shoes have enough room for their toes.

STUDY SESSION: IS BAREFOOT BETTER?

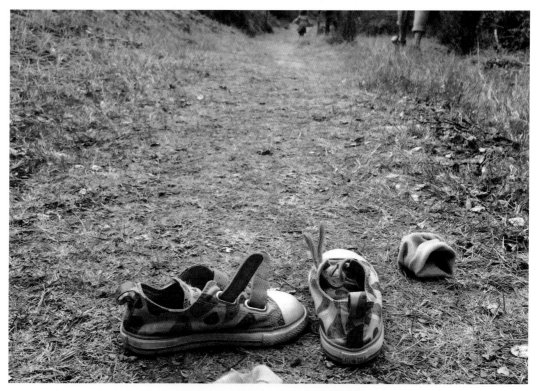

Is barefoot time really necessary for human children? Are conventional shoes *that* bad? We've only recently begun to realize humans have more "natural needs," so this question is new to researchers.

Several studies on adults show that a lifetime of being habitually barefoot seems to result in wider feet, higher arches, fewer toe deformities, and more flexible feet compared to those habitually shod. A similar study of children suggests many of these differences can be seen by age six to ten. Shoes do change the feet! It's hard for studies to separate the effect of age from the length of shoe-wearing time, because age also changes the shape of the feet, but researchers have noted that barefoot time might be most influential during the growing years.

Researchers have compared how foot anatomy works while barefoot with foot anatomy in both flexible and stiff shoes. They found that stiff shoes hinder a lot of the way feet move when walking. They note that if barefoot walking offers the best opportunity for foot development, then flexible shoes should be recommended for healthy children in general.

They've also found a difference in the performance of motor skills (like balance, jumping, and sprinting) between habitually shod children (six to eighteen years old) in Germany and habitually unshod children in South Africa. Those with more unshod time had better balance and jump length while aged six to ten years, but not better sprinting times, although the unshod children's sprints were measured mostly on natural terrain, whereas the shod children sprinted over hard indoor flooring.

It's hard to state unequivocally that being barefoot is better than wearing shoes, because shoes protect feet from unpleasant natural and human-made stuff on the ground. But it's clear that always wearing shoes leads to different feet and different ways of moving. Striking a balance between barefoot time to develop stronger feet and flexible shoes when you need them most is a conservative approach to get the best of both worlds.

Hollander, K., J.E. de Villiers, S. Sehner, K. Wegscheider, K.M. Braumann, R. Venter, and A. Zech. "Growing-up (Habitually) Barefoot Influences the Development of Foot and Arch Morphology in Children and Adolescents." *Scientific Reports*, August 14, 2017.

Wolf, S., J. Simon, D. Patikas, W. Schuster, P. Armbrust, and L. Döderlein. "Foot Motion in Children Shoes: a Comparison of Barefoot Walking with Shod Walking in Conventional and Flexible Shoes." *Gait & Posture*, January 2008.

Zech, A., R. Venter, J.E. de Villiers, S. Sehner, K. Wegscheider, and K. Hollander. "Motor Skills of Children and Adolescents Are Influenced by Growing up Barefoot or Shod." *Frontiers in Pediatrics*, April 25, 2018.

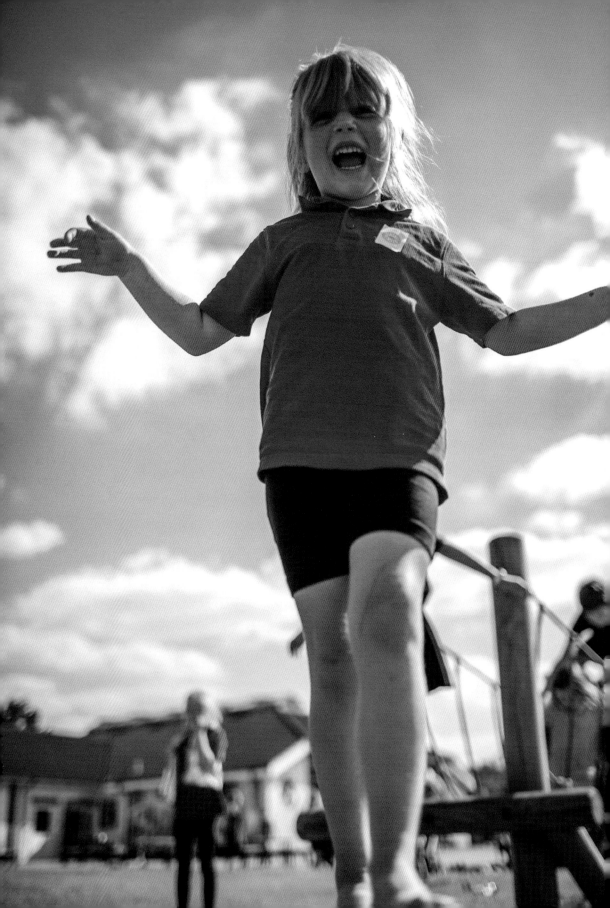

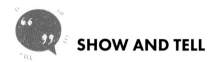

SHOW AND TELL

Mine and my friends' kids spend barefoot time outdoors from spring to autumn. Grounding nature walks take place whenever we get the chance and are such a treat, as they really lift the spirits of everyone involved and boost our energy levels (adults included!). My three-year-old almost never wears shoes during summer anymore, and for England that is almost unheard of! My friends now allow their kids to go barefoot whenever it is safe to do so and understand the benefits for their developing bodies. The kids now run barefoot after school in the field and playground and the head teacher is going to trial my recent suggestion for barefoot time for all children at school when we go back after summer break. Barefoot time can catch on quickly and is such an easy way to get more natural movement into the kids' day. They love spending time barefoot on the trim trail and encourage the other kids around them to try too! We're educating others and leading by example.

—Emily Doe

CAN THIS OUTFIT CLIMB A TREE?

It's not always easy to see which body shapes an outfit allows. Here are some movement tests to consider before buying or making an outfit.

Can both arms reach overhead comfortably? In addition to maximizing movement at the shoulders, make sure that the entire "chest" of the outfit doesn't rise up toward the face when the arms lift overhead—that's a sign of inflexible clothing. Ideally, the arms should be free to fully move out in front, overhead, to the sides, and behind.

Can you bring a knee to your chest? Stretch a leg out to the side? Look for pants with legs that are loose or stretchy enough to allow full hip and knee bends, not only front to back, but also out sideways (see how legs might need to move for a climb on page 127).

How will the outfit shape work with the environment? Is any part of the outfit oversized or flowy? Loose fabric can catch on things that you try to pass over or around. How will catching affect your movement? Will the material fray easily if it gets caught?

Do these shoes help or hinder? Will these shoes stay on my feet or fall off as I move my legs up the tree? Will they grip to the tree bark or will they slip?

This principle can be applied to any movement. Below are a few more examples, and if your child has any specific movements they love, like leaping, for example, consider how clothing might impact those moves.

Can this outfit squat? Does the waistband cut into your middle when

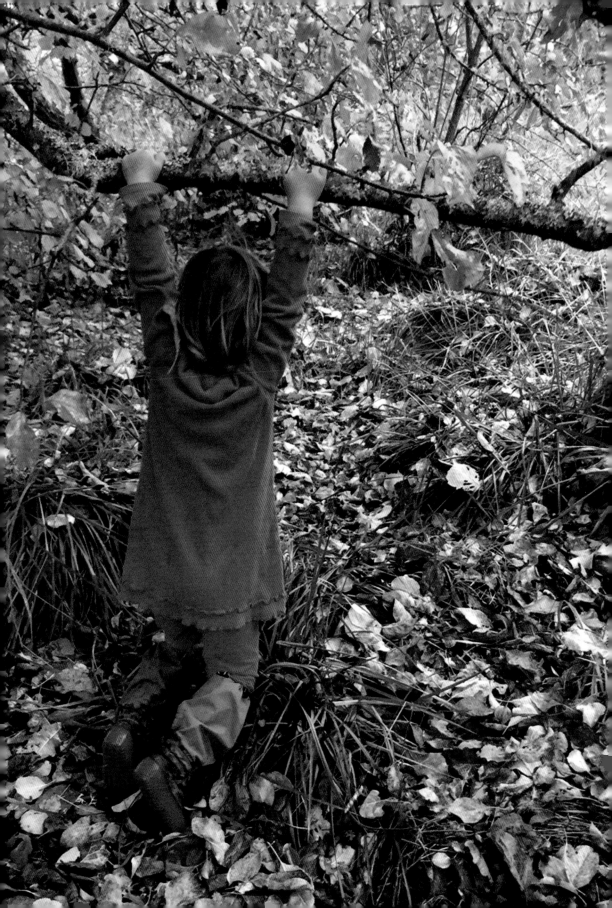

you bend forward, squat, or kneel (do you feel like the tree on page 4)? Are the legs loose enough or stretchy enough to allow full knee bends?

Can this outfit invert? If you've got a tumbling kid, be on the watch for clothes that fall down (or is it up?) disruptively into faces and around arms and knees when the child is upside down. Select clothing that is flexible but stays in place—like more fitted shirts, and leggings or other flexible pants with cuffs that stay down at the ankle. If you have a modest monkey who loves dresses, pair them with leggings or shorts underneath to keep them cartwheeling, climbing, bar-twirling, and crawling. You can also teach them the trick of tying up a skirt with a hair elastic to keep it out of their face when they're upside down.

Can this outfit walk a mile? Do any parts of the clothing feel scratchy or uncomfortable? How about if you kept your parts moving repetitively inside them for an hour or more?

Evaluating the movement abilities of an outfit might take a little practice at first, but soon it will be a quick and simple process that takes less than a minute. Better yet, the discussions and movements you have when trying on clothes will become part of your child's knowledge base. Not only will they learn how to test and select clothes themselves, but more importantly, they'll learn that movement (or a lack of movement) is something that can be chosen or not. "Sedentary" becomes less of a default.

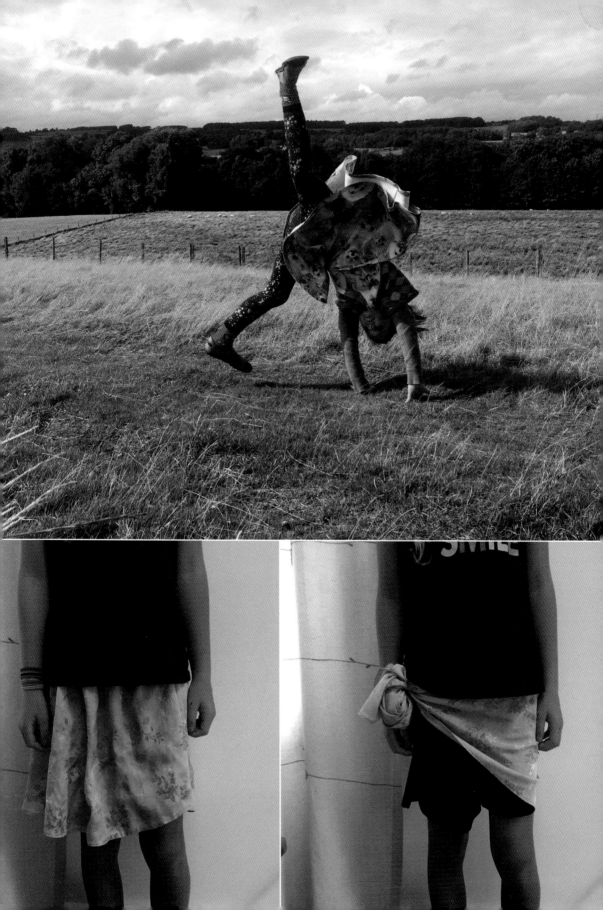

ADORNMENT IS DIFFERENT FROM APPAREL

Both of my kids get dressed in apparel every day, but only one of my kids is what I call an adorner.

This is the kid who could dress herself at eighteen months, spent years covered in paint and marker tattoos, cut her own hair, mulls over the right outfit every morning, covers her head and hair in complicated wrapped scarves, taught herself to braid and otherwise style her hair, and loves sparkle and makeup. Her way with her wardrobe is not about fashion (it's almost the opposite of following a trend) and more about expressing herself through what she puts on her body. Both my kids have a personal style, but for the adorner, her body is a canvas and decorating it is an art—*her* art—to be created and worn each day. Humans have long decorated their bodies—there might even be some sort of adornment-trigger in our DNA—and accepting that her need for adornment might be primal helped me when the three-year-old adorner wanted to start wearing high-heeled shoes.

Before I had kids I assumed that the desire for heels came from seeing a lot of people or images of people in high heels. But I don't wear them, our friends don't wear them, and even the picture books we read together don't automatically put every female character in high heels. Still, high heels are essentially wearable foot art, so there's no wonder an adorner would be naturally drawn to them. They quickly change the look and feel of an outfit and the body wearing it.

But, have you ever tried walking, running, climbing, cartwheeling,

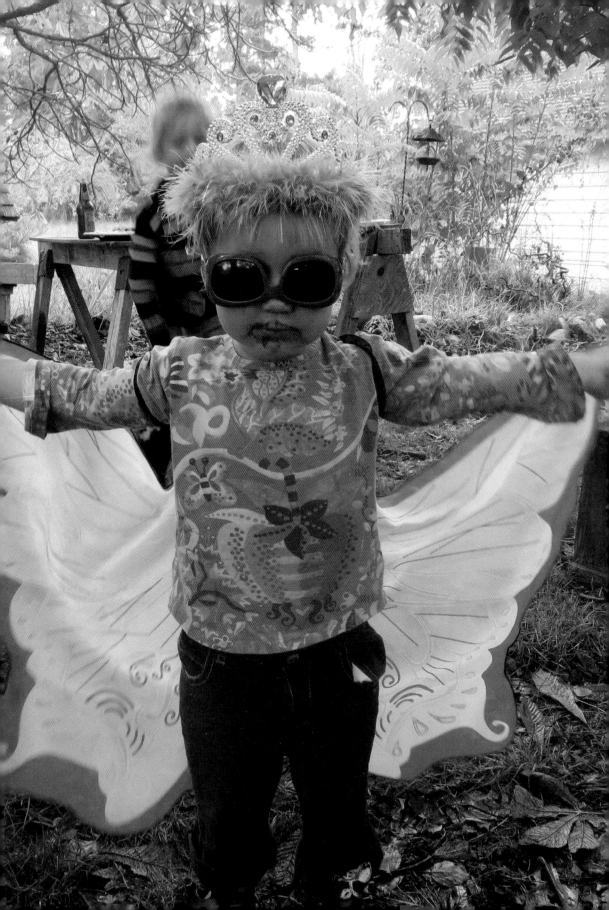

balancing, or vaulting in high heels? Unless you're in *Charlie's Angels*, high heels do *not* help you move more. They actually limit your movements—and not just of the feet and leg parts. They tend to keep a whole body in place because they can be so hard and even painful to get around in. I realized we needed to come up with a way to decorate her feet that was more dynamic than heels in order to meet this kid's needs for adornment and movement at the same time.

When she was younger, foot adornment came in the form of stickers, ribbons, paint, and markers. Even mud shoes were part of her play. As she got older, we moved on to beaded, crocheted, and once straight-up ribbon-from-the-trash-can foot jewelry. In short, style autonomy matters to all kids but some will need more assistance in making the leap to a more dynamic wardrobe, especially when there are way more "sitting around" options than there are "dynamic wardrobe" options.

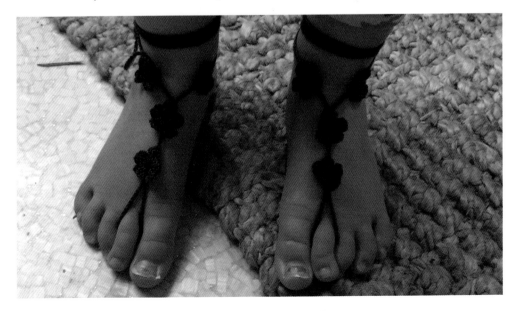

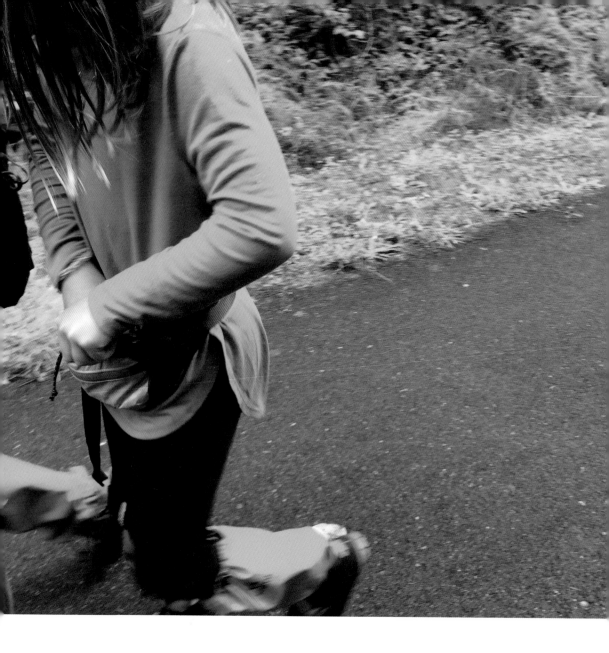

Long walks are part of our family culture, and one thing that has made them more exciting for our children and more enjoyable for us is letting them carry their snacks. Once they were around six and seven, I liberated myself from having to dig into my bag any time they wanted to deal with energy or boredom issues through a snack. They also end up moderating their eating better when they can put their eyes and hands on what they've got left. Butt/hip packs make light loads for littles, and they offer an alternative to heavy shoulder loads.

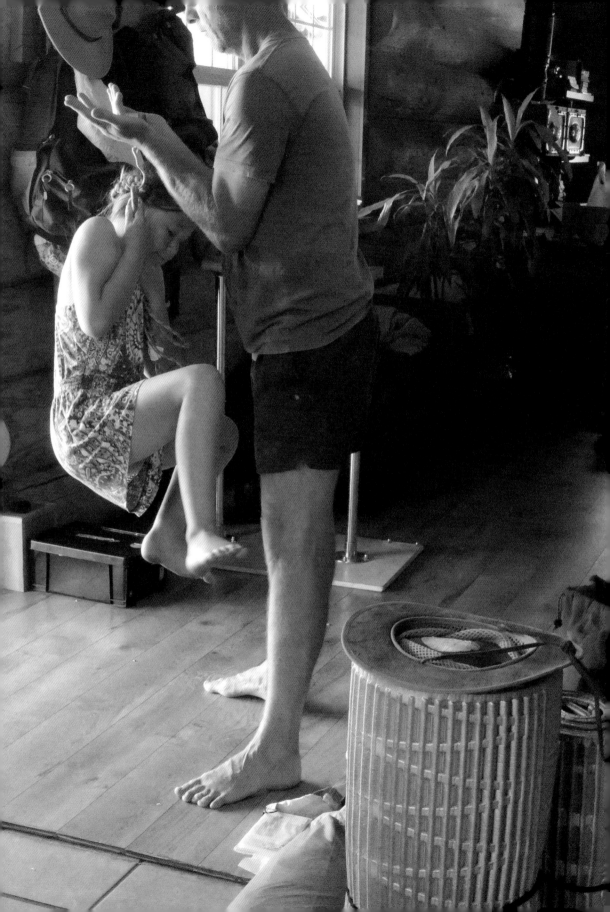

We use a luggage scale to figure out the weight of our backpacks and, for fun, the weight of our kids (to calculate how heavy to make their backpacks).

What's the ideal pack weight? It's not clear. Recommendations tend to be "X% of bodyweight,"—typically 10–15%—but that's not always helpful. Are you talking about carrying a bag for thirty minutes distributed throughout a mostly-sitting school day? Walking for a number of miles? Uphill or downhill? What type of bag? Is weight the best variable to compare against, or is it muscle mass? How do lessons in form or carrying experience affect the body and how it works while carrying? When it comes to outdoor adventures, I have my kids carry what they can, in a way that allows for good form AND a positive experience while also letting them dab a toe (or two) into their grit. This 70-pound/31-kilogram kid carried about 12 percent of her bodyweight the first, steep uphill day. She also likes to distribute her pack weight by putting her "snack butt pack" around her waist. I took on 3 pounds/1.3 kilograms of her load for the second half of day two (more steep uphill) and all of the seven miles down. I plan my bag weight assuming I might also need to handle some of theirs for part (or even most) of our adventure. This amount worked because of her muscle mass, hiking experience, and practice carrying lighter loads over a variety of distances. In short, we practice child-led, parent-attentive pack-carrying.

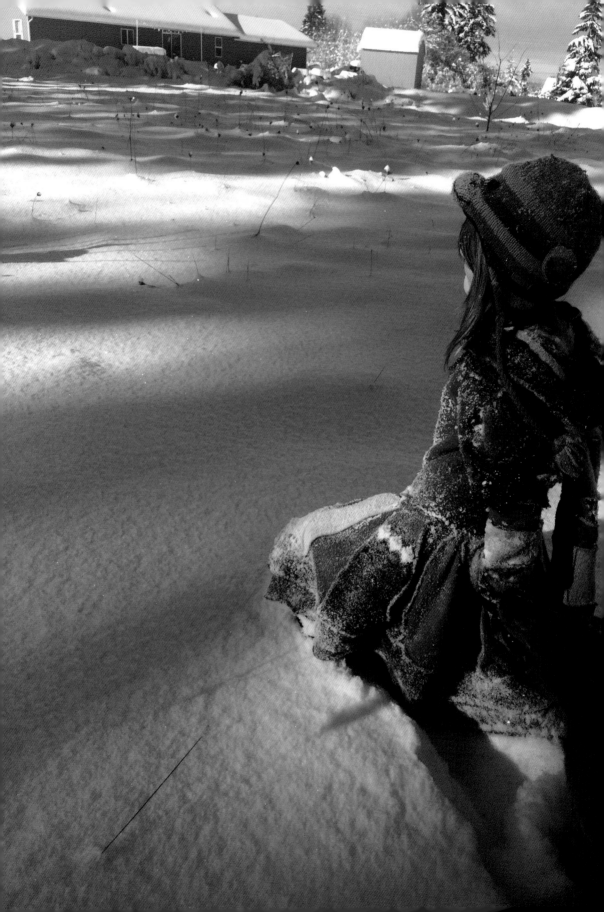

We were fortunate to have a preschool-kindergarten nature school in our area. We looked over their clothing guidelines (see page 122) and sourced the recommended raingear. My three-year-old adorner promptly rejected the black synthetic pants because they were a) pants, b) not colorful, and c) didn't feel "right" on her body. She loved the school but hated getting dressed in the "uniform," which made for miserable mornings. I just couldn't figure out how to put her into all-weather (including snow) nature school without rain pants—until I happened to flip through an issue of *National Geographic* featuring a shepherding culture living high in the mountains. There, upon the pages, was a picture of a shepherd girl leading her animals through knee-deep snow while wearing a colorful, body-length wool dress. It was an "A-ha!" moment. Humans have been in all sorts of weather without "gear" for thousands of years; they used wool! My crafty friend repurposed wool sweaters to create a colorful felted wool dress that fit over the adorner's base-layers of clothing, keeping her warm, waterproof, and stylish for years. Our family often selects wool clothing as our snowgear because it's flexible, sustainable (when produced in a regenerative and humane way), and easier to find at thrift stores. And bonus: wool doesn't melt like the plastics in synthetic materials do when a spark from an outdoor fire falls on it!

A NATURE SCHOOL'S GUIDE TO WINTER CLOTHING

Olympic Nature Experience, a nature school in Washington State, shares some of their insights into how to dress for success. Find out more about them at olympicnatureexperience.org and find them on social media at @olympicnatureexperience.

Helping your child dress comfortably for inclement weather and modeling a positive attitude and curiosity about the weather ("I wonder what fun things you will do in the rain today?") are the two best things you can do to set your child up for success for time outside, no matter the weather.

Initial investment in the right clothes will last your child throughout an entire season and often beyond. This gear can be used thoroughly and often resold or passed on multiple times.

Below are some tips we've generated based on our Pacific Northwest weather; most are adaptable to where you are too!

GENERAL TIPS:

Know that anything your child wears could get muddy or wet, and be okay with it. Having extra clothes packed can help keep you relaxed about these matters (store extras in their school bag inside an extra plastic bag, which will keep clothes dry in case of wet or muddy backpacks).

Layers, layers, layers! Many thin layers can be more comfortable than one thick layer and are more flexible for heat regulation. Tuck shirts into pants and socks over pants to keep body heat circulating near your core.

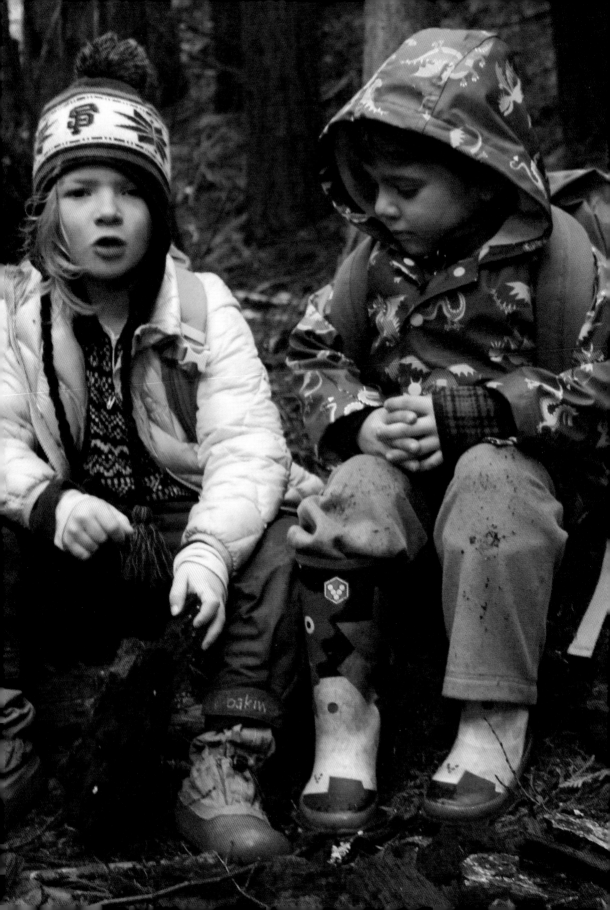

Avoid cotton during wet/cold months. We always recommend rain pants on the outside to keep your child warm and dry.

Make sure their clothes allow lots of movement!

When possible let them try on gear to make sure they are comfortable and enjoy it. Some children will be very particular about what it looks like, and others will care solely for feel.

SHOES AND SOCKS:

Use "water shoes" combined with wool-blend socks for extra warmth/comfort during the spring through fall or in drier climates; they can be put in the washing machine with other clothes, and their thinness allows for excellent traction and versatility.

Look for winter or rain boots with the most flexible sole and as little heel as possible. Mobility of the foot allows for naturally generated warmth.

Wool-blend socks are a necessity in the winter; they'll keep children's feet warm even when wet. Also, an extra pair in the backpack can also work as hand-warmers if the need arises.

HEAD AND NECK:

A well-fitting wool or fleece hat is best, and we've found neck warmers to be preferable to a scarf so they don't get tangled. Neck warmers can also double as a hat.

MITTENS AND GLOVES:

Gloves often go missing! We recommend having multiple pairs of gloves/mittens for your child, and to pack extras. Thin polyester gloves/mittens, thick wool mittens, and thick ski gloves are examples, but make sure you label every glove (especially if gloves also go to school). They will get them wet, no matter how waterproof they are, and you will need an extra pair on the wettest days.

UNDER LAYERS:

Wool blends, polyester, or fleece against your child's skin make a great "base layer." No need for fancy gear: long johns, pajamas, or other thrift-store-found items can work great as base layers! If your child's core stays warm, the need for gloves is minimized, and adding small layers on top of a base layer leaves a lot of room for them to adjust their temperature throughout the day.

PANTS:

For younger children, **stretchy waistbands are ideal** for easy (autonomous) and fast bathrooming.

Rain pants are a crucial layer and are great for being outside when it's wet or windy. They also keep your child comfortable even when it's not raining, because the ground will be cool and damp. Rain pants and suits can be very effective if properly waterproofed. During very rainy weather, rain pants are often better than snow pants; snow pants can absorb water and rarely have ankle cinches. Pick pants with an ankle closure (Velcro, elastic, cord and toggle) to cinch the pants tight over boots to keep water out.

COAT:

A solid fleece coat with a sturdy, proven rain jacket on top are ideal. This keeps the warmth in and rain and wind out. It is crucial that the waterproof coat has a system for cinching at the wrist to keep water out.

TREATING RAIN GEAR:

The current thinking says to put rain gear in the dryer to improve its waterproofing, but old advice was to avoid drying rain gear. Check with your rain gear maker or local outdoor store.

If waterproofing ability begins to fade or to ensure extra-strength waterproof ability, you can treat your gear with a Durable Water Repellant (DWR). These come in sprays or washes and you can find them at your local sporting goods store or online.

By observing and listening to your child and their experiences, you'll find the right balance for them. Our school's philosophy is all about helping kids connect to nature, and we want to make sure clothing is not getting in the way of the connections they'd like to create.

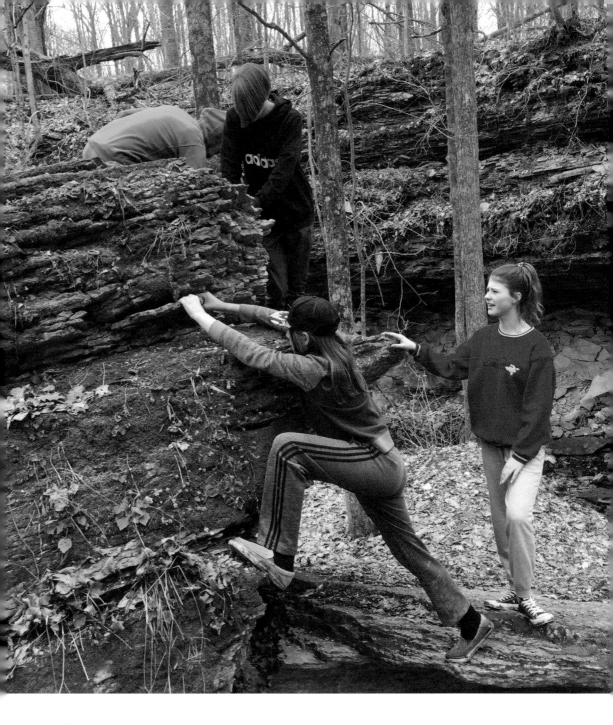

A body that can otherwise do a move won't be able to overcome clothing that cannot. Think about the movement potential of an outfit and teach kids to make sure their clothing won't prevent movement experiences.

A NATURE SCHOOL'S GUIDE TO WARM WEATHER GEAR

Many parents write to me about how impossible getting more nature/outdoor time feels when it's really hot outside. Diona Williams, MA, M.Ed, is the owner of Out Back Learning LLC in Sierra Vista, Arizona—a part-time preschool that focuses on the growth and development of early childhood through nature-based play with children and their families. Below are some of Out Back Learning's tips for gathering gear that supports nature play in hot weather.

The most helpful gear when it comes to hot-weather nature time is a clock! Avoid the hottest part of the day (10 a.m.–2 p.m.) when scheduling your outside time. Seek out nature or outdoor play in the many hours before and after this midday period.

Grab a hat. A wide-brimmed hat or baseball cap is portable shade and creates a cooler environment wherever you go.

Sunglasses! Protect wee eyes from light (and wind, in some cases) with kid-sized sunglasses (if you can find ones with UV protection, great!). Keep them from getting lost by adding a strap that allows them to stay around the neck when kids take them off to look at a bit of nature up close.

Wear long, lightweight pants and shirts. Light, breathable clothing can keep skin out of the sun by covering the skin. Look for materials that ventilate well and add these as layers over T-shirts or shorts that work best in covered or shaded areas.

Umbrellas. Not only for rainy weather, umbrellas are also great for sun-blocking and can quickly create a cooler environment while kids are walking, drawing, or having snack time outside. Create a resting spot with a beach umbrella if your outdoor space doesn't provide much shade.

Pack a sitting blanket or towel. The ground can radiate heat, making sitting next to impossible without some sort of chair. Fortunately, a blanket or towel is a lightweight solution that fits all terrain and can make taking a seat on hot, gravely, or rough surfaces more comfortable.

Finally, remember that sunscreen and a water bottle are essential apparel in sunny weather. Forgetting these is like forgetting to put on pants—your hot-weather nature time outfit just isn't complete without them!

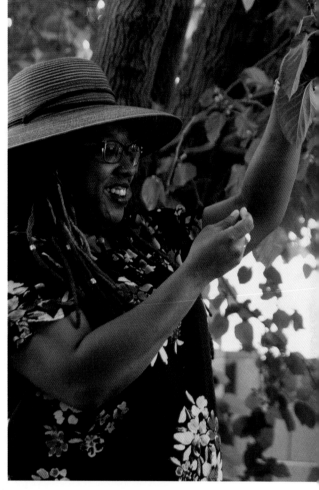

For more inspiration and education, find Diona Reese Williams online at dionnareesewilliams.com.
Facebook: Diona Reese Williams (Education Consultant Agency), Out Back Learning LLC
YouTube: Diona Reese Williams DRW
Instagram: @drw_dionareesewilliams, @outbacklearning2019

IT'S NOT THE CLOTHES THAT MAKE THE (HU)MAN, IT'S MAKING THE CLOTHES THAT DOES

Just as adornment has primal roots, making, or the art of crafting, is a primal skill. Until very recently, humans, including children, made their food, clothing, and tools by hand rather than buying everything ready-made by machines and other people. While we've gotten rid of the need for making most of our necessities ourselves, we haven't entirely gotten rid of the movements and skills that go into making, so schools fit making lessons (arts and crafts) into their curriculum.

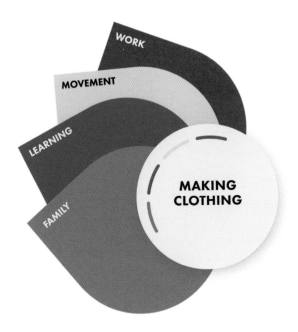

TASK: MAKING CLOTHING
NEEDS MET: FAMILY, LEARNING, MOVEMENT, WORK
BONUS NEED MET: *Adornment*

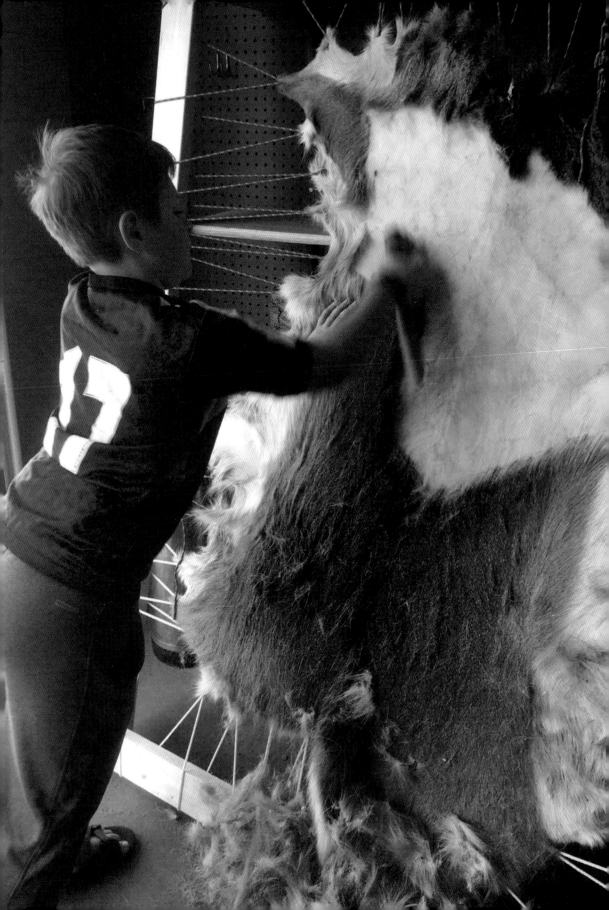

But the crafts kids make at school don't usually have a purpose beyond the process of making them, and they tend to be pretty much disposable straight away. For better stacking, we've found apparel to be a natural way for our adorner to move her making muscles while learning crafting skills, how to work for what she needs, and expressing her style. Sewing, mending, weaving, knitting, crocheting, processing animal hides, and making jewelry can give crafts a real-life context and deepen a child's relationship with meeting their needs for clothing and décor as well as their fine-motor movements. When children are young, making time can also be great family time, and once they're older, these skills become what they reach for in their free time.

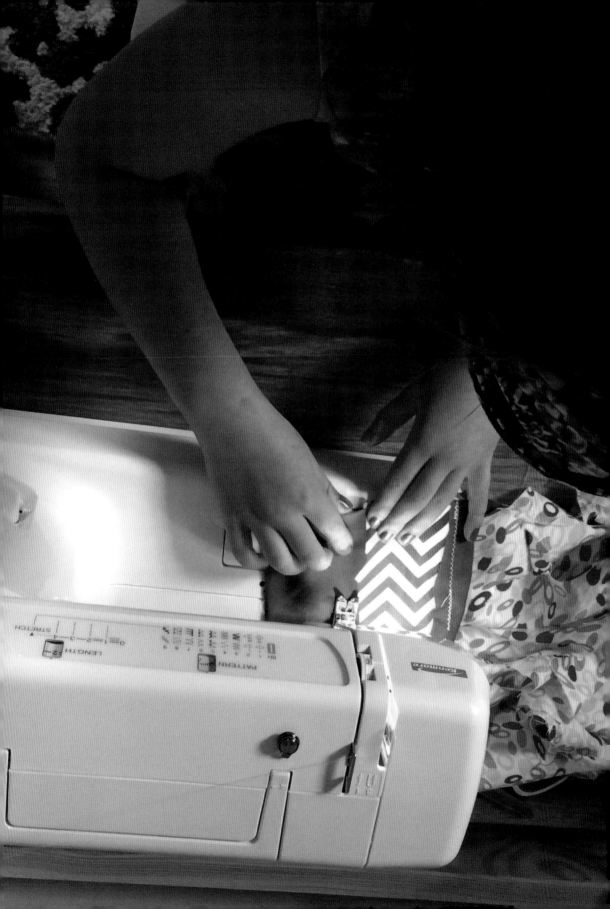

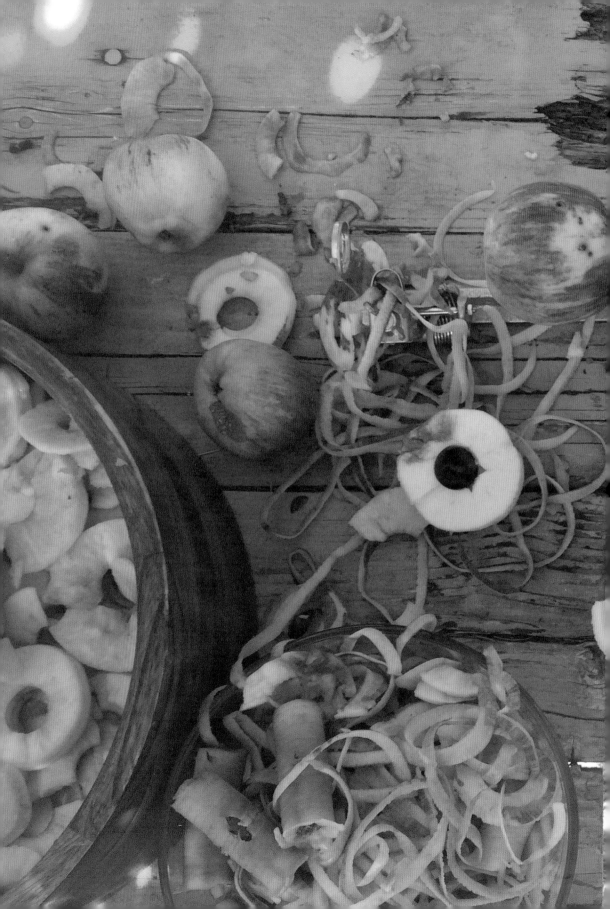

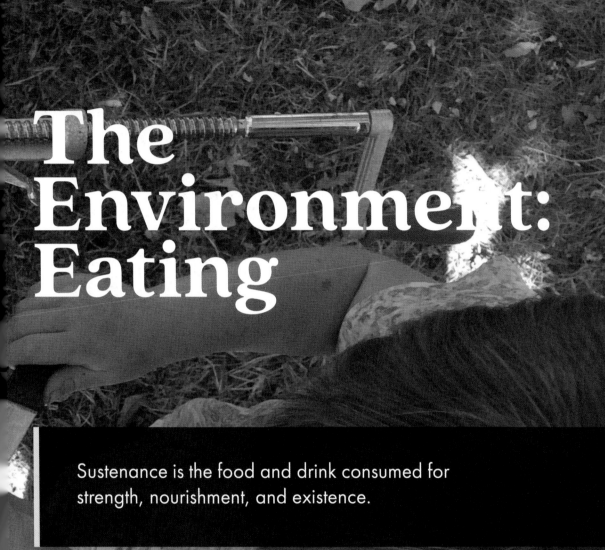

The Environment: Eating

Sustenance is the food and drink consumed for strength, nourishment, and existence.

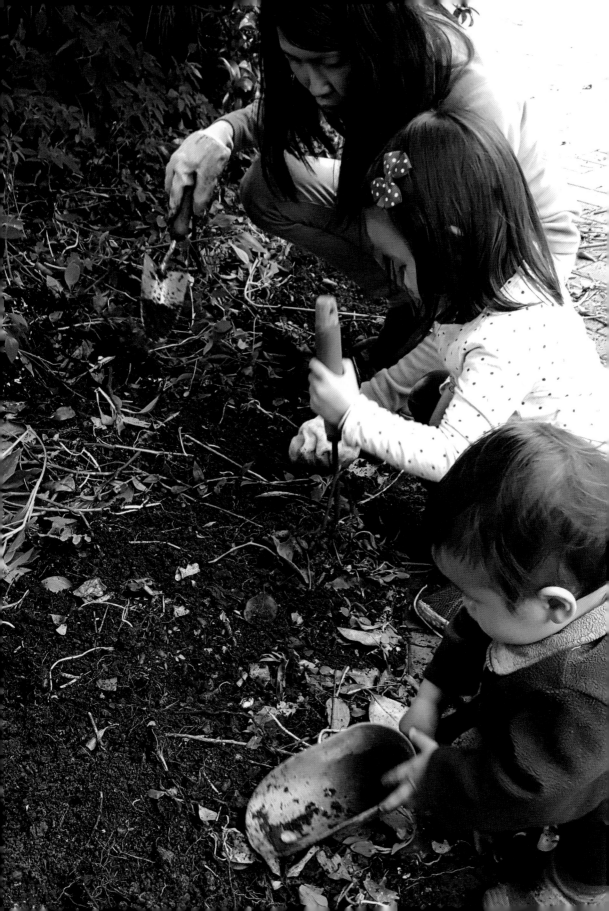

The Cooking Container

chapter four

C hildhood takes forever. Now that I'm a grown-up, time seems to fly, but I can still recall the feelings I had when I was a kid. Would I ever grow up? When would I get to do what *I* wanted to? When would I learn what I needed to (so I could then do what I wanted to)? WHEN WOULD I GET TO DRIVE? Childhood felt like an eternity, and it turns out my senses weren't that far off: humans have a relatively long juvenile period compared to other large mammals.

Why do humans have such long childhoods? There are a few theories as to why the kid-phase of being a human came to take such a long time, most of them centered around our big, energy-expensive brains and the reasons these brains might have evolved as they have. But what is clear is that learning to feed ourselves adequately takes a really long time. In our closest relative, the chimpanzee, youngsters produce as much food as they consume by the time they are around seven years old; in forager cultures, human children are not self-sufficient until they are at least fifteen (see Kaplan in this section's references for more).

For thousands of years, eating took a lot of human power—human movements necessary to search for, gather, grow, cultivate, and process plants and animals into food. Eating well also required equally abundant nature literacy: the education necessary to develop the ability to "read" things like animals and plants, seasons and landscape. Every human, even young children to the best of their abilities, contributed their personal human power to feeding themselves, and thus the "food system" for each person was fairly small. You and your community did the labor directly for the stuff you ate, and all of that movement happened in nature.

Currently there are humans on the planet who live in hunter-gatherer communities, and while their modern practices are diverse and not exactly what they were thousands of years ago, the way their families subsist in nature gives us an idea of how much movement (and nature, learning, family, community, and play) is stacked with food. Take a minute to imagine just some of the food moves kids used to be involved in each day: walking and climbing to locate food; the fine-motor movements of tool-making (bows and arrows, cordage for traps, basket-weaving for carrying and cooking); the tool-using movements (squatting, digging with sticks, rock/spear throwing, net-casting, sprinting); the hauling of water, wood, and heavy foods (an animal carcass or a basket of tubers); and the repetitive pounding of ingredients between heavy objects to process them into something edible. And think, for a moment, about the chewing (jaw and face-muscle movements) we'd all need to be doing if it weren't for blenders and mills and steak knives breaking our food down into smaller bits! All kids, even hunter-gathering kids, eat soft foods as they wean, but agriculturists (that's us, who eat foods selected and produced by agricultural practices) seem to keep soft foods going throughout our lifetime.

Food moves these days look quite different for many. Grocery markets are full of food that's already grown, harvested, and processed for us. We can get into a car and grab a meal, already cooked, without even standing up. Other people and machines perform the entire spectrum of human food movements on our behalf—from finding something edible to gathering to processing and even to *breaking it down into tiny pieces* (smoothie to go!). The matter of feeding ourselves was the environment that used to move us the most, but it now takes very little personal movement, time in nature, or knowledge of the plants and animals we consume. Eating today hardly requires any chewing!

But here is some great news: Though we've gotten rid of our food movements, eating continues to occupy a tremendous amount of our time and energy as we think, plan, and buy (or work to buy) our food. Our life is still full of food, and food is still the gigantic environment it's always been. We know that food used to be the primary source of kid and family movement and of movement in nature, so we know where to go looking for more of that movement. When it comes to choosing where to add more movement next, the food system is the ripest environment. We have so many moves to discover and recover!

STUDY SESSION: READING NATURE

Children learn in many different ways. While direct teaching is one way, learning happens mostly when they observe, imitate, participate, and play.

It's always been that way. "Hunter-gatherer" (H-G) is a term that applies to many culturally diverse groups. Despite their diversity, there are similarities in how children growing up in H-G societies learn to eat.

Some research has focused on their learning experience. In general, modern H-G infants are worn on their parents, who are often gathering food. They begin observing the human-food relationship right off the bat. Throughout early childhood, food moves are central to their play in the form of using play tools to play-harvest and play-trap. Groups of children climb trees (an element of gathering honey, fruits, and nuts) and hunt small game. What's "stacked" about H-G food play is that it results in actual food. The kids' tools work; it's just that the kids aren't super skilled at using them yet. While the play-gathered food offers fewer calories than the children expend gathering it, it contributes to their overall needs. By the end of middle childhood (about age eleven) children can adequately *collect* food.

As kids get older, they start to learn, through immersion but also through direct teaching, the carving and weaving "making movements" necessary for making simple tools and traps, as well as how to hunt with them. Older kids join in with groups of adults going out to hunt or gather, and by immersing themselves with adults of varying skill and experience, they eventually graduate into being food-securing adults.

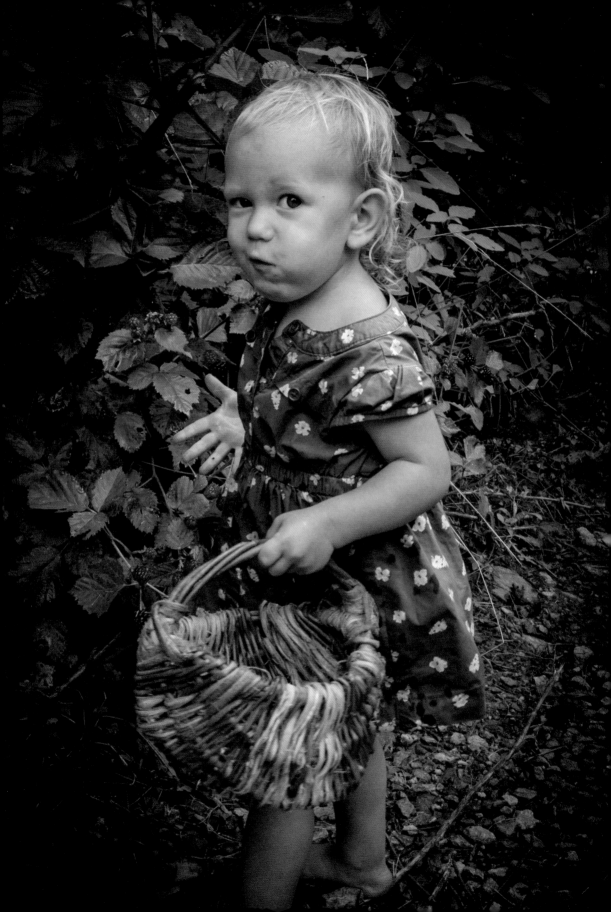

All the while, children are learning to "read nature"—animal signs and behaviors. According to one anthropologist group writing on the San (the indigenous H-G groups that make up the first nations of southern Africa), "Walking around the bush reading and interacting with nature is the most important activity of any day." Just like regularly putting books in young kids' hands is part of learning to read, getting outside to walk and interact in green spaces is how children develop fluency in nature.

While you or I might not be required to spend a portion of our day walking through nature for the interaction or knowledge that activity provides, if you talk to your local farmer or those doing a large portion of your food moves for you, it's likely they still do. Observing soil, water, weather, and plants is essential if you want to be able to eat; farmers and gardeners often teach their children how to do this too, whether directly or by example. Food security cannot be boiled down to being able to make enough money to buy it; food security goes much deeper. It includes food moves that are intrinsically nature moves, and these are the natural human movements that got us here and are still required. Reading nature is as important to humanity as we've made reading symbols on a page.

When it comes to figuring out how to infuse your life with more food movement, I think we're actually quite close to this type of learning. Our kids are exactly the same as H-G kids; the brains and bodies of all children, any place and any time, are wired to take in copious amounts of information about how the society around them works and how they work within that society. They are wired to convert those experiences to play and to develop proficiency in them. Thus our kids regularly engage in "food play" via toy food, toy kitchens, and by

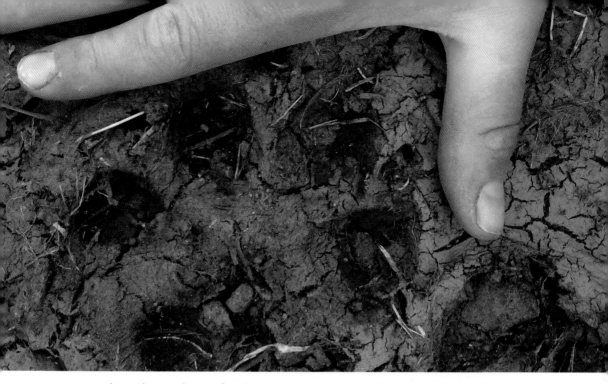

mimicking their culture's food moves in game-style (anyone else used to play "grocery store" and pretend to be the checker? What about playing "drive through"—anyone? Anyone?). Their period of natural food-keenness therefore makes them experts in our culture's sedentary food moves. By unstacking the food from the food play, we squander this valuable phase of their development and let them become proficient at eating food but ignorant of enormous amounts of food-nature knowledge and food moves.

Gallois, S., R. Duda, B. Hewlett, and V. Reyes-García. "Children's Daily Activities and Knowledge Acquisition: A Case Study among the Baka from Southeastern Cameroon." *Journal of Ethnobiology and Ethnomedicine*, December 24, 2015.

Imamura, K., and H. Akiyama. "How Hunter-Gatherers Have Learned to Hunt: Transmission of Hunting Methods and Techniques among the Central Kalahari San (Natural History of Communication among the Central Kalahari San)." *African Study Monographs Suppl.*, March 2016.

Lew-Levy, S., R. Reckin, N. Lavi, J. Cristóbal-Azkarate, and K. Ellis-Davies. "How Do Hunter-Gatherer Children Learn Subsistence Skills?: A Meta-Ethnographic Review." *Human Nature*, December 2017.

SNACKTIVITIES AND MECHANICAL NUTRIENTS

If you search "snacktivities" on the web, you'll likely find images of fun, edible crafts to make with kids—mostly treats. I'm not sure if the idea was to add food to art or art to food, but I think the idea goes something like this: kids like to craft and kids like to eat, so why use paper and glue when we can make a snack playful and kill two birds with one stone?

If the role of snacks is to fill a belly, then snacktivities go a step further in the needs they meet: in addition to dietary nutrients, you're also providing a "making" opportunity for the same calories, and that making can also be playful. A snacktivity is therefore a stack! It combines "making," food, and play, so it meets more than one need at the same time—no matter what foods you're cooking.

I like the snacktivity concept because it reveals that we're willing to do more with our food than just eat it, and that we're even used to the idea. Even better would be *snacktive* tasks that add more than art and play to our food: we need to add back the movement, nature, and learning that once came with all foods.

Earlier I explained how movement works like a dietary nutrient (movement bends your cells, which in turn convert that bend into chemicals, which affect that cell's behavior). Each movement bends our cells uniquely; each movement makes different nutrients (more on that in chapter seven). There are tons of movements to be done for food (food moves!), which means that food can provide many different dietary nutrients and many different mechanical nutrients.

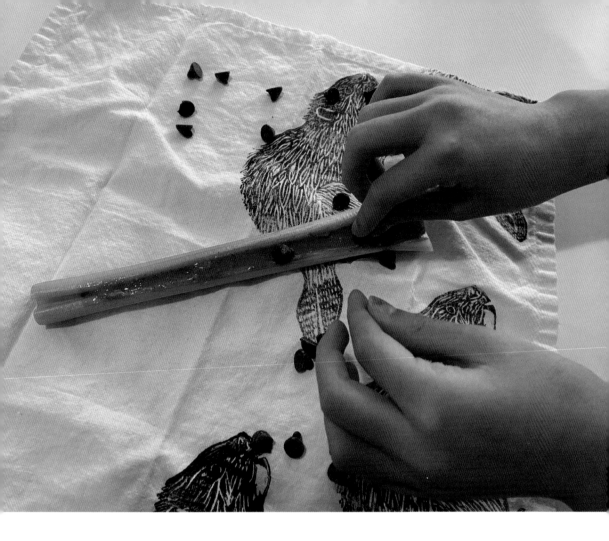

Consider an apple. It has dietary nutrients that include energy, carbohydrates, fiber, vitamin C, vitamin K, and potassium. Some of its *mechanical* nutrients include the tooth and jaw movement to bite and chew it; the climb, bend, or squat to reach it; the walk to and from the apple tree, the carrying of it home in a load with other apples. These are examples of mechanical nutrients that come from doing the labor it takes to convert an item of the earth (an apple, in this case, but the movements differ depending on the item) into something that provides dietary nutrients. The mechanical nutrients are created by *how we are moved by the apple*.

Now, if we cook down that same apple—softening it—the dietary nutrients are the same, but we've changed the mechanical nutrients. Chewing isn't required as much as slurping, which provides fewer mechanical nutrients to the jaw and the other face muscles and tissues that would be moved by chewing. If we open a jar of applesauce from the store, then the mechanical nutrients reduce again. We don't need to do any climbing, bending, walking, or even chopping for the same dietary nutrients…only slurping movements. The apples in applesauce no longer move us in a walking, climbing, bending, reaching, chewing, carrying way; they move us in a drive-to-the-store-and-slurp-them-up sort of way.

The diets provided by the landscapes humans come from have shaped human anatomy and physiology, and kid and grown-up bodies still depend on these dietary and mechanical nutrients for full health! Humans have tinkered enough to figure out how to pull dietary nutrients out of various sources and bottle them up so doses of nutrients are available *unstacked* from the more nourishing food source. Now we're doing the same with movement—trying to get the bends and squishes our bodies need through minutes of daily exercise, which is a very unstacked approach.

If we want to get kids and families moving more, then we have to add more movement time to the day, and for most of us, the only way to do that is to add movement to the periods of time we're already using to meet other needs. We all need to move, eat, *and know about how and where food comes from*, so an ideal way to meet all these needs is to apply the principle

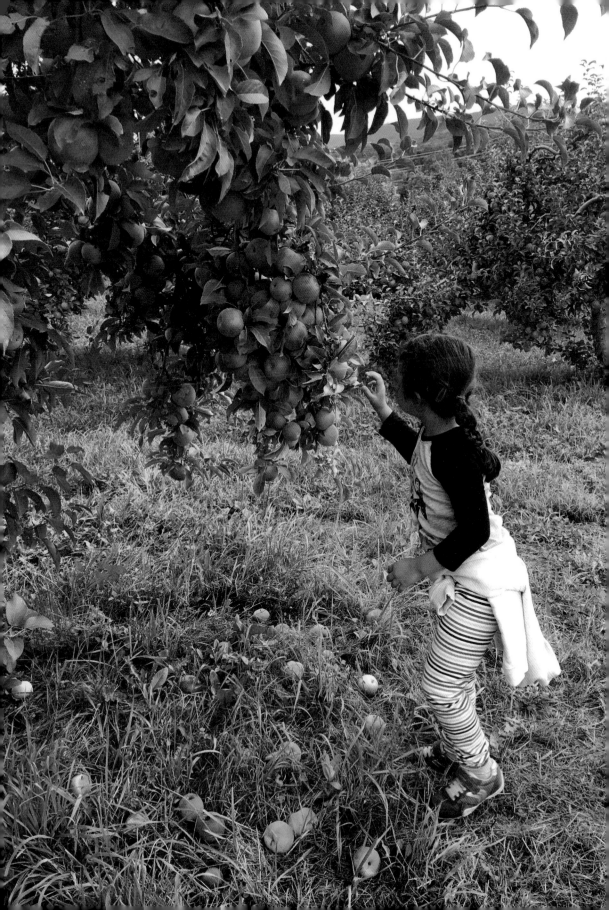

of movement permaculture (the layering of movement with dynamic tasks that have been used by humans for millennia) to the food system. THIS IS WHERE WE GET SNACKTIVE, FOLKS!

You can't go wrong in your search for the mechanical nutrients associated with food, because food moves are so abundant. They range from the bigger-body movements of finding, growing, foraging, harvesting, and processing, to finer movements found in food-related tool making, as well as the movements that go into making, cooking, and even eating (chewing!). We haven't been doing most of them, so there are SO MANY PLACES you can start getting more family food moves. Just pick a food move, any food move!

MOUTH MOVES

There is more to food than what's contained within it. The forces created when we chew plants and animals play a role in how our body works; chewing, ripping, tearing, and swallowing provide the necessary mechanical stimulation to develop strong, optimal anatomy and function of jaws, face and throat muscles, vocal cords, Eustachian tubes, sinuses, throat glands…the list goes on. A fun experiment to try with the kids: Have them put their hands on the sides of their jaw and have them bite down lightly and then more forcefully. What do they feel? Have them put their hands on their temples and repeat the process. Chewing exercises our faces!

Think of the foods kids eat as a sort of playground for the face muscles and tissues. We might have been selecting foods for their energy, vitamins, and minerals, but are most of the foods kids eat soft? If yes, then this is like moving on a playground that only has a sandbox. A kid can play a lot in a sandbox, but it's not going to offer a big variety of movement. Instead we can choose foods that take a lot of jaw and face movement—strong biting (carrots, whole apples, nuts), tearing (jerky, dehydrated fruit), and processing (any food that takes a lot of chewing to break it down). Adding more mouth moves to a lunchbox is like adding a set of mouth monkey bars, a tongue tightrope, and a swallowing swing set to the eating playground. You're packing more essential movement into a meal.

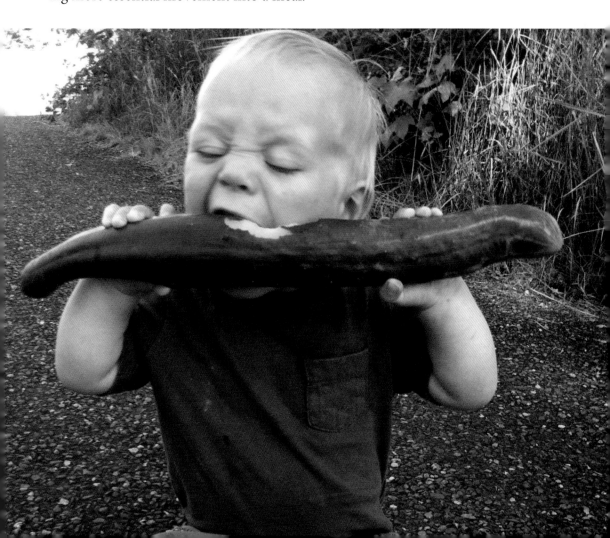

BABY'S FIRST FOOD MOVES

Some of the first movements for baby mammals, including humans, are *food moves*—complex mouth moves of the jaw, tongue, palate, throat, and face muscles—that draw milk from the breast and into the belly. Some bodies don't produce milk, some bodies cannot gather it, some societies have been set up to make the production and the gathering of human milk problematic,

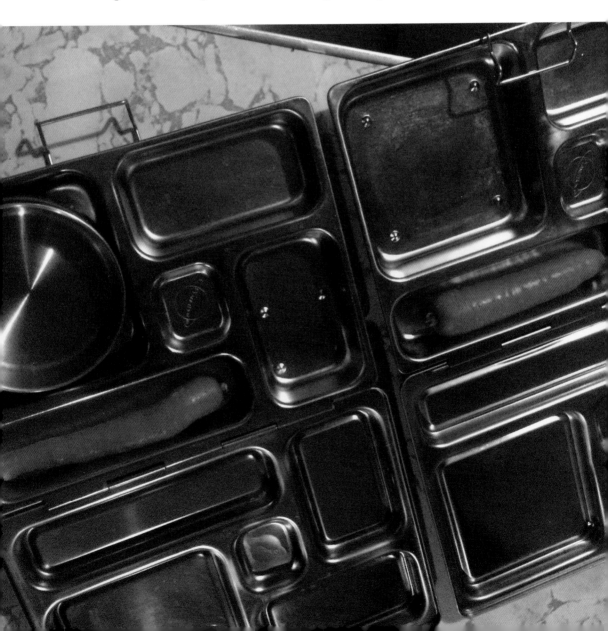

and how we've set up our individual lives might be influencing our children's earliest food moves. There is *no* judgment of anyone's individual situation here—I'm simply detailing the phenomenon of our first mammalian mouth movements and why they might matter.

We say mammals suck, but the way a baby's mouth works at the breast is much more like a farmer rolling their fist down a goat's teat. Feeding at the breast moves more than mouthparts; in fact, breastfeeding is a well-choreographed face workout. Like any workout, it builds and strengthens our muscles, bones, and connective tissues to make us better able to do those specific movements. Feeding at the breast offers more than the dietary nutrients found in breast milk—there are the mechanical nutrients too, *not found elsewhere.*

Breastfeeding and bottle-feeding can be touchy issues, especially for new parents, and I want to reiterate that I am *not* casting judgement about whatever way your particular baby is being or was fed. We can celebrate bottle-feeding for its positive impact on countless lives. Still, we can explore the movement differences between breastfeeding and bottle-feeding to recognize the limitations of (and maybe improve) our technologies, as well as keep in full view the ecological effects of the biological processes behind how human babies feed.

In many cases, feeding from a bottle, whether it contains breastmilk or formula, has been associated with nipple confusion (not knowing how to move the mouth on a breast) and too-early self-weaning, which is associated

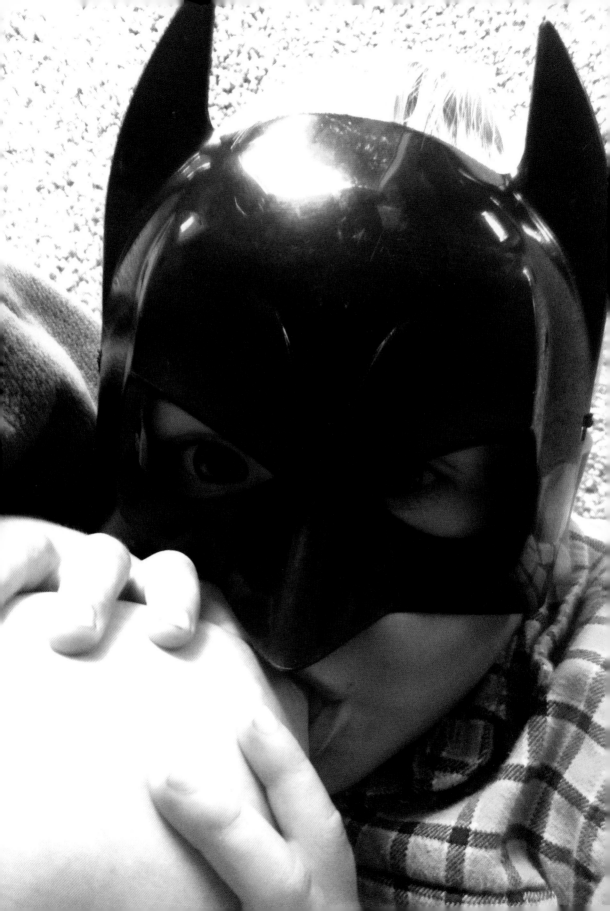

with ear problems, respiratory infections, gastrointestinal issues, chewing and speech issues, dental issues, and other oral habits. Researchers are considering the role movement is playing.

So far, there seem to be two things going on. The first is, feeding at the breast requires more movement than feeding at the bottle. According to research on healthy, full-term infants that looks at "sucks per minute" a baby performs, bottles require fewer sucks, breasts require more, and mixed feeders (babies with skill in both) move somewhere in between. It's simple mechanics: a bottle lets the milk flow for less work. Babies can get used to that amount of work, and when they're given the harder task of breastfeeding, their bodies haven't been trained to do it.

The second is, bottle-feeding doesn't only mean *fewer* food moves, it means *different* food moves. Again, it's simple mechanics: while both feeding styles use muscles in the head and neck, breastfeeding uses different muscles and moves different bones than bottle-feeding does. If infant suckling is a playground, then the bottle features fewer pieces of, and entirely different, playground equipment than the breast does. Feeding is still completed either way (and thank goodness for that!), but still, certain movements have become unstacked from the feeding process.

Human bones, similar to trees, are shaped by how they are moved throughout our lifetime, and human jaws have been changing shape. As the bulk of humans have gone from H-Gs to agriculturists to post-industrialists to living computer-based lifestyles, their skeletons reveal how the loads of each of these times differ: our jaws aren't being coaxed into shapes that can hold all of our teeth anymore. Evolutionary biologists and dentists have seen increased prevalence of poor tooth and bite alignment.

Teeth are a different tissue from bone—they're less malleable and therefore less responsive to the mechanical environment as they form. Their genes send them growing in a genetically determined way, even if the bones they are growing within are too small to hold them. This creates tooth crowding and malocclusion issues that take dental, orthodontic, and sometimes surgical interventions to correct. This situation is one example of "mismatch theory," a theory that explains that the environment human genes have been exposed to for tens of thousands of years is an integral part of how human bodies work. When there is a relatively fast change to the environment, human genetics often can't keep up.

Researchers have been looking at the movement environment created by breast, bottle, and non-nutritive sucking (thumbs and pacifier), because it is these *literally formative years* that most greatly influence the shape of our skeletons. Human mouths and faces have been shaped by the breastfed playground for so long, it's likely that our physiology currently has a built-in requirement for suckling-at-breast movements as part of how our anatomy forms and goes on to serve other functions (like chewing and breathing). However, we now have bottle-feeding technology, and dental-related technologies and therapies, so we could argue that humans don't actually require breastfeeding. On a baby-by-baby basis, it works! We do need to consider the phenomenon scaled up to a massive population, though, and the amount of resources pulled from the earth that go into these technologies. Feeding at the breast is simply the most *stacked* version of early feeding; it offers the dietary and mechanical nutrients babies need in a low-impact, portable way that helps everyone move with more ease.

TABLE MOVES

"Table moves" are those whole-body positions we've choreographed to go with eating.

While humans gathering together around a meal is a fairly universal phenomenon, somewhere along the line, eating, for many of us, started requiring *special dining furniture*.

If we think about mealtime positioning as a food move, then how does eating an apple at a table differ from munching the fruit while sitting on the floor? I'll get into furniture in general in chapter five, but basically, positioning yourself on the floor, and getting down onto and up from it, requires a lot more movement of the ankles, knees, hips, and spine.

Our culture closely associates eating with sitting on chairs around a table, but I've found mealtime is a perfect opportunity to quickly increase a family's food moves just by changing up or simply moving away some of the furniture.

You can create a permanent low-table eating arrangement (see more in chapter five), but you can also immediately and easily spread out a cloth (like a sheet, blanket, or tablecloth) on the floor and eat picnic-style for more

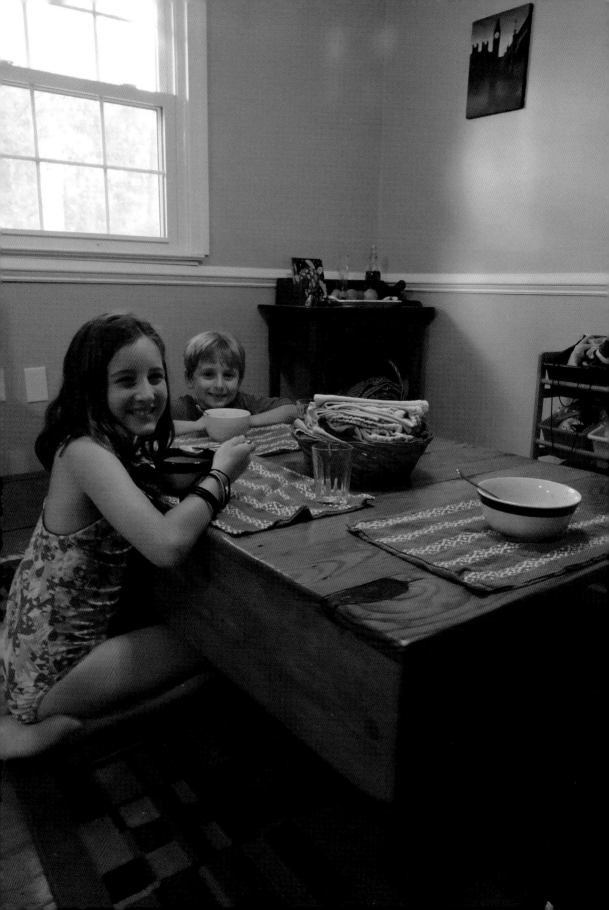

movement. Note: kids love the novelty of this, and novelty is often what makes moments special. To add a dose of "nature," throw that cloth onto a balcony, porch, yard, or nearby park and take the meal to a place you can hear the birds, feel the wind, and stretch your legs out on the ground. Many organizations recommend families sit together for dinner as a sort of daily bonding, and I agree that this connection is so important. I just challenge the idea that this connection can only happen sitting in a chair at a table.

But wait: do we even need to be sitting at all? No! I've stacked more family time, movement, and nature into our meals by taking our breakfast and/or dinner to go. Sometimes we make a portable breakfast and walk to school (you can drive partway and walk a distance that works for your family) or make dinner food that we can take for a stroll. P.S. There is benefit to paying attention to the food you're eating as well as to the fact you're chewing it, so know that you can always stop to chew and swallow or take small breaks for eating in between your adventures.

KITCHEN MOVES

Grating, cracking, chopping, peeling, mashing, grinding—these are just a handful of the "making food" movements found in kitchens everywhere. Until the very recent emergence of convenience foods, these movements were done by many people, every day.

Convenience foods save us time; however, since children still need to move, learn about the food system, and spend time with their families, convenience

BABY FOOD TO GO

Feeding doesn't only move the baby, it moves the body providing the food too. One of the questions I get asked most often about infant-feeding is how to do it so it hurts less. Sitting in a single position over and over again, whether it's at a desk or in a car on a long drive, can make the body ache after a while—that's a signal to get moving! Similarly, in Western cultures we almost exclusively see infants being breastfed or bottle-fed in a single position—the adult relaxing back, resting deep into some kind of furniture, cradling a horizontal infant (and don't forget the feeder's rested face and serene smile; never once looking haggard or horrified after dropping a smartphone onto the baby's head). But what if we took that meal to go?

You can take a breast- or bottle-feeding session out of the chair or couch and to a place where you can stretch your hips open on the floor or upper back against a couch edge. You can lie down on your side and stretch out. Once you've worked through any feeding issues and the baby's latch is sturdy, add some of your own movement back in. Anthropologists note one of the ways breastfeeding differs between modern H-Gs and Western populations: H-G mothers nurse while cooking, sewing, and out in the bush gathering. I went into motherhood as an experienced hiker and able to carry a load. Thus, I didn't think twice about bringing my young infants with me (as H-Gs all over the world do!) and fed them deep in the woods or trailside near my house. Sometimes even while continuing on foot. Personal note: "Boob walking?" was a common inquiry from my still-nursing toddlers looking for their version of a shot of trail mix while out on an adventure. You can add the movements you feel comfortable with, but

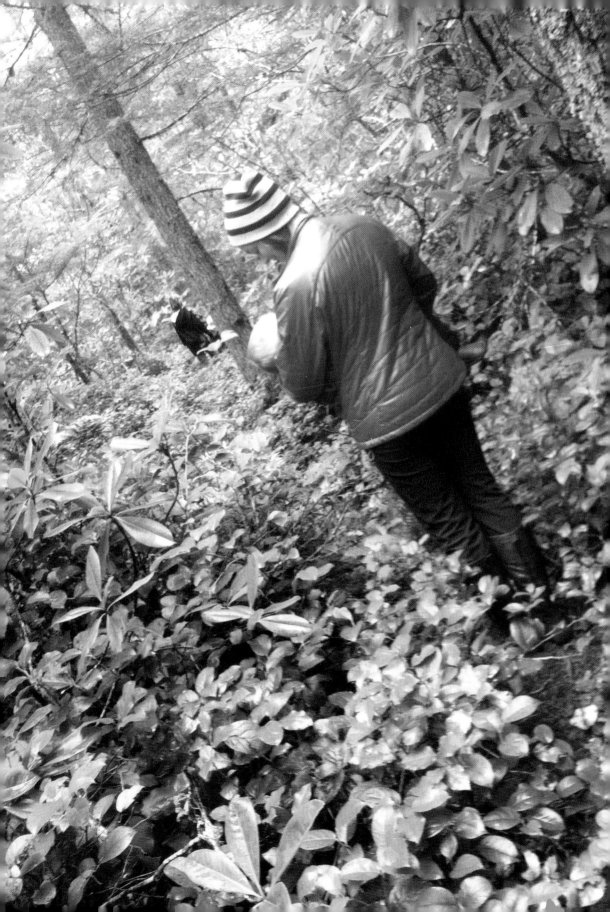

my point is this: part of why we keep feeding time so sedentary is due to how infant feeding is modeled in our culture—how it looks in books, on packaging, and in commercials. That's truly just a way one group of people is doing it.

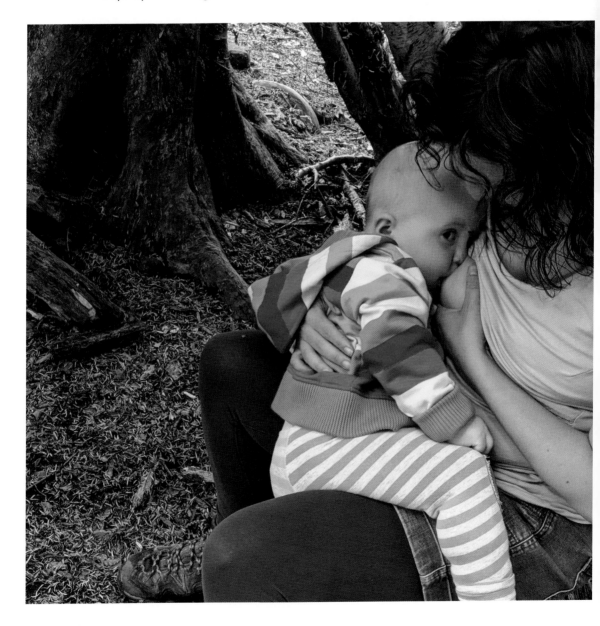

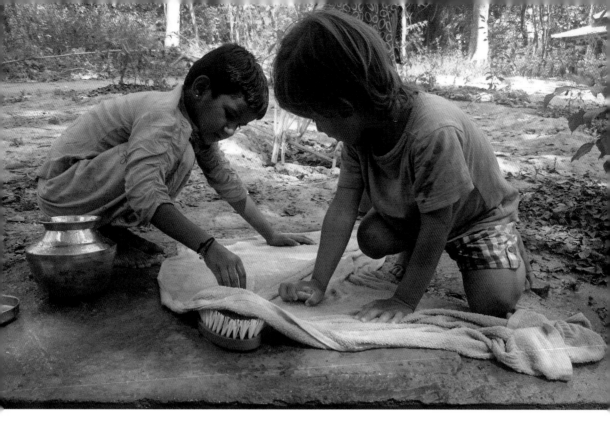

foods wind up not saving us much time at all. Kitchen moves can be a stacked, whole-family way to move, learn, and connect through nourishment.

I remember my great-grandmother used to pull out pots, lids, and spoons when I was very, very young. As I sat on the kitchen floor with her bustling around, I was already learning to move in the kitchen—no special toys needed to be purchased. As I got older, I was able to get more involved in productive moves. From cracking eggs to grating veggies to grinding coffee, kids like food prep work (and they really like food prep tools).

Our family likes to use prehistoric "snacktivity tools" including rocks (for shelling nuts), mortar and pestles (for mashing whole spices), digging sticks (for gathering potatoes), and the ground (for sitting). The adult-sized surfaces, chairs, and tools that fill our houses don't work as well for little bodies and can actually increase things like falls and injuries as children learn to cook. You can arrange your kitchen so it's more accessible to the wee people in your life. While it might pose a design challenge to set everything down to their level, remember it's impossible for them to set themselves to your level. And, P.S. You'll find yourself moving more to get to that lower level, now that things are no longer conveniently at waist-height (stack)!

Some helpful tools:

- Children's size whisk

- Small grater

- Small mortar and pestle

- Hand grinder

- Low table (and remember that working on the ground is an ancient practice for human bodies of all sizes! The ground most easily "fits" a child's body)

GROCERY STORE MOVES

Dynamic diets are a human baseline. Humans have always needed to walk daily for their food and water, and many humans today still do. Even for those of us who no longer *need* to move for food, it's always an option.

As a parent, feeding my kids is always on my mind. It's easy to start feeling overwhelmed at having to figure out meals and a grocery list, to take a trip to the grocery store, cook it all up, and then wash a billion dishes. So I decided to enjoy the process—and stack it with a walk.

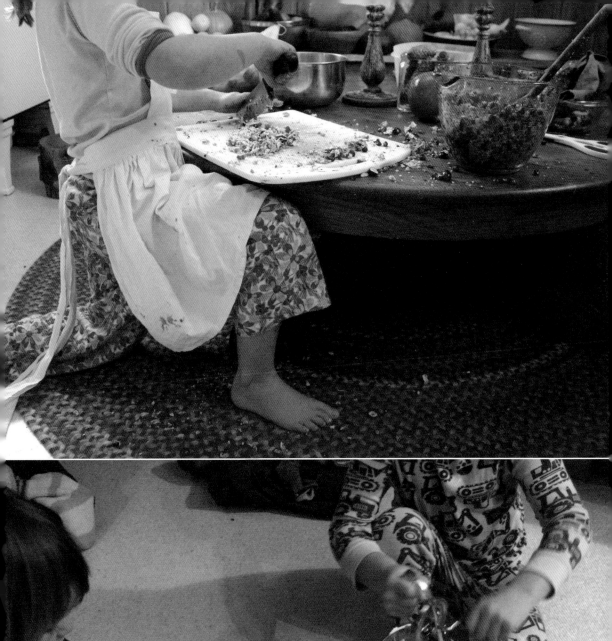
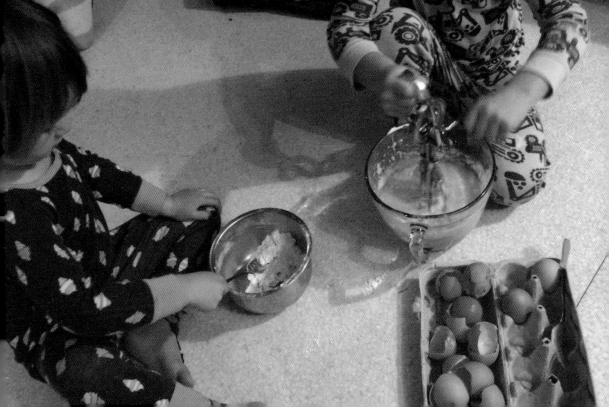

NATURE KITCHEN

There are a ton of ways to set up dynamic kitchen and cooking spaces outside to add some nature to your kitchen (or some kitchen to your nature!). If you have a balcony, you can spread a cloth on the ground and do all your prep outside. If you have a little more room, you can add a freestanding fire pit, a barbecue, or a camp stove. If your region allows, you can set up a ringed cooking fire—or you can travel to a park or other community area where you can flex your outdoor cooking muscles.

Kids have been cooking their own food on a fire for thousands of years and this activity makes for a nutrient-dense meal of knowledge and nature-rich, dynamic food. Some of my favorite campfire cookbooks are: *The Campout: Inspired Recipes for Cooking Around the Fire and Under the Stars* by Marnie Hanel and Jen Stevenson, *Feast by Firelight: Simple Recipes for Camping, Cabins and the Great Outdoors* by Emma Frisch, and *Dirty Gourmet: The Best Camping Food for Your Adventures* by Emily Nielsen, Aimee Trudeau, and Mai-Yan Kwan.

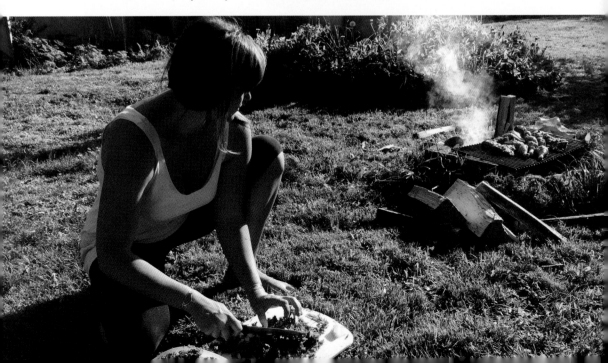

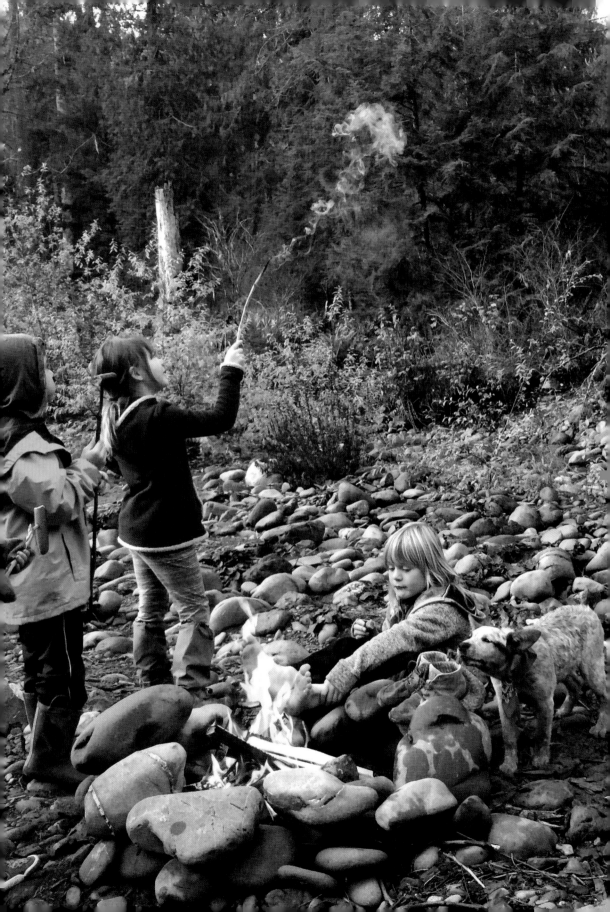

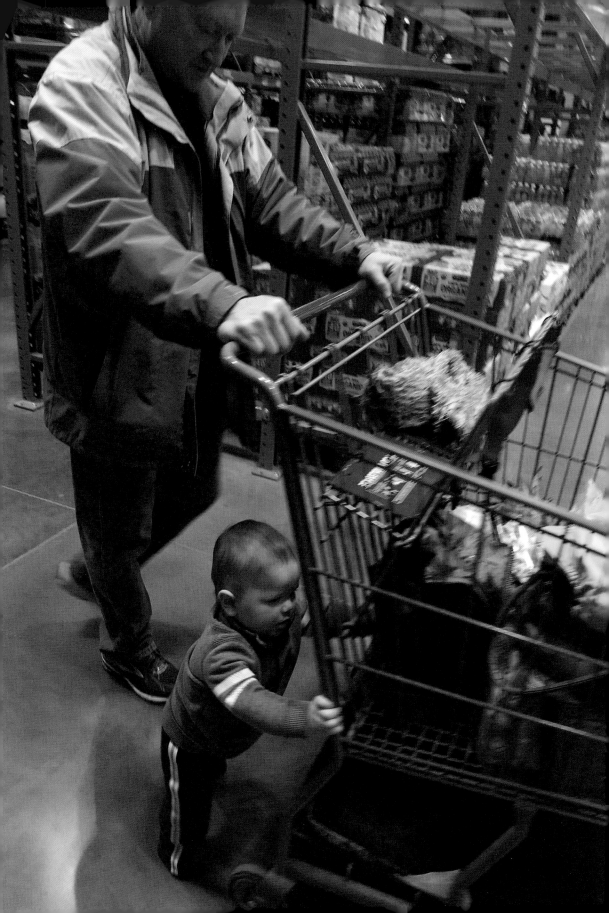

For decades, fitness and health magazines have suggested we park our cars as far from our destination as possible to get more steps. My more stacked version of this is a regular family walk to the store for our food. You can walk all the way there or drive partway and walk the rest of the distance for an hour of outdoor movement for everyone. It can also be time for a family chat, game playing, or whatever style of connection you're looking for. More frequent walks to the store can also mean lighter loads and lots of carrying for even more movement. The movement doesn't stop when you get to the store; you can find more of it *in* there by selecting your foods with care. Dieticians often point to "whole" foods as a more nutrient-dense dietary choice—foods that have not been chemically refined or processed and have no additives or preservatives. Similarly, I recommend *actual* whole foods—the same foods recommended by dieticians, only not pre-chopped, pre-shelled, or pre-cooked. They are literally more "whole." They contain not only more dietary nutrients but the mechanical ones too. Whole eggs, whole spices, nuts with their shells on, whole fruits and veggies all need to be moved before they are eaten (they're often cheaper too). A kid's kitchen moves start with the ingredients in the home, many of which come directly from our grocery store choices.

GROWING MOVES

The magical transformation of a seed to a plant is so important for humans to understand, and you see this lesson show up in schools across the world. Many young children get to learn through actual experimentation—planting a seed in an old milk carton they've filled with dirt, watering it, and moving it from window to window to learn about the effects of sunlight. Other children will learn about this process through pictures and words in books, theory and quizzes.

Our existence depends on growing plants, and humans all over the world are struggling to understand this connection. Alarm bells should be ringing at the fact that in our particular culture, fewer and fewer citizens, especially fewer and fewer of our *child*-citizens, share the experience of growing plants, especially in a hands-on-learning way. Growing food is, at its most foundational level, about security, sovereignty, and survival, and we are becoming less aware of how to do it. We've not only outsourced our food moves, we've outsourced our food knowledge! Good news: you can stack a plant-science lesson with growing moves and get a mealtime payoff.

And the list of gardening payoffs grows further. There is currently a huge resurgence of community gardens that provide food-growing space, information, and support, which is ideal for people who are just starting out or don't have room at their own homes. Empty lots are being converted back to green spaces that stack the need for more local and nutritious human food with riches for pollinators and birds.

Growing moves can be simple even if you've never grown anything before. It doesn't require expensive gear or a lot of space. You can sprout beans in a mason jar, start a flat of microgreens, or have a few pots of fresh herbs growing

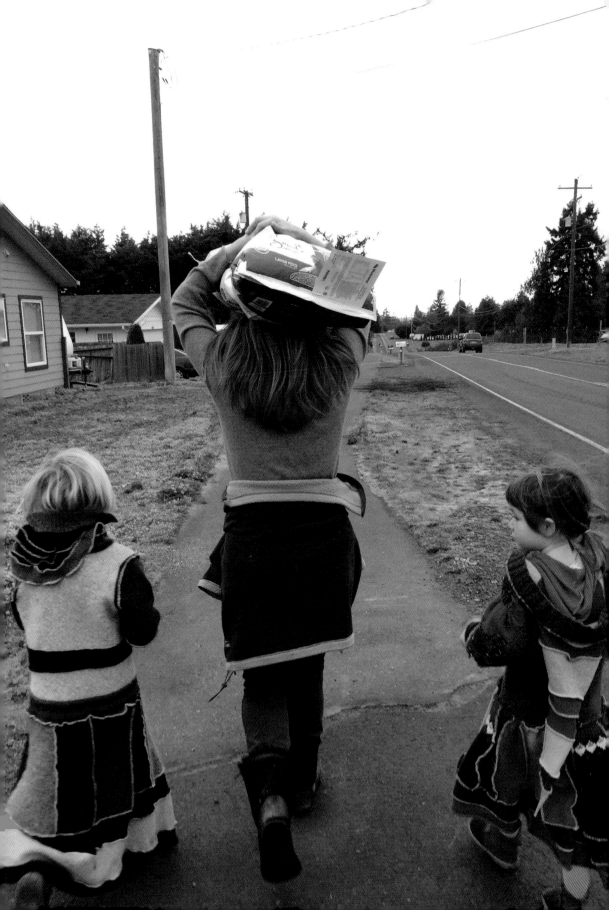

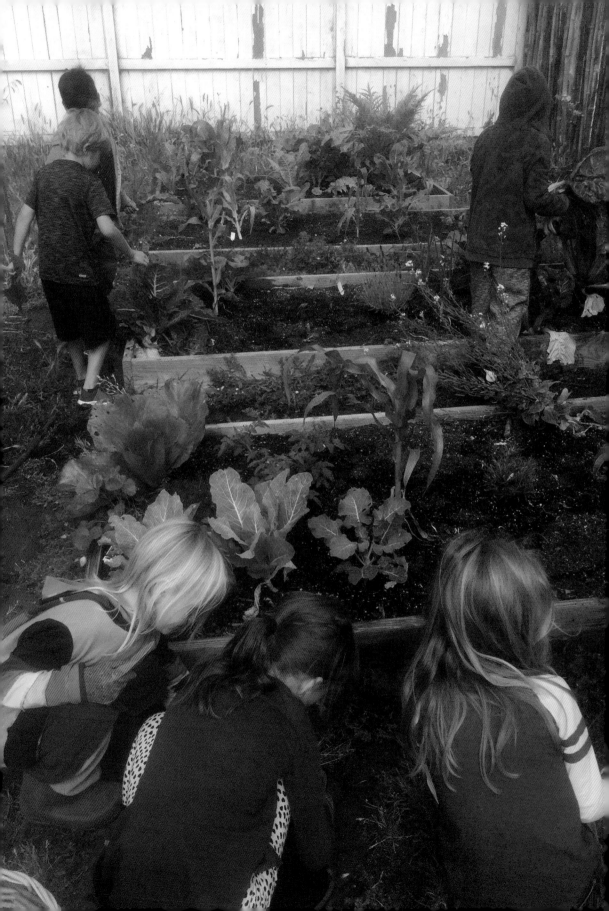

in almost any dwelling. You can have a balcony overflowing with tomatoes and spinach, or you can smother the grass in your yard and create some veggie beds instead (read the book *Food Not Lawns* or visit foodnotlawns.com for more on how to do that). It's an enormously scalable project, and no matter what scale you're growing on, it can be immensely satisfying for a child to have produced even the smallest part of their own meal.

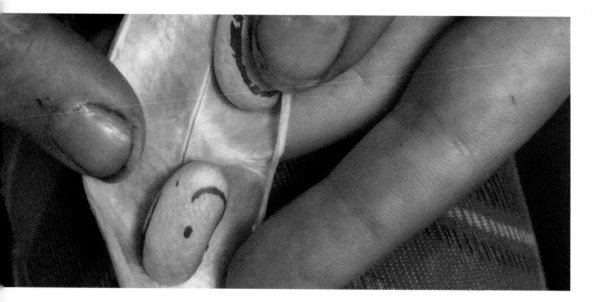

FARM MOVES

No matter where you live, there are almost certainly food producers within reach. Some farms are industrial, but there are still many smaller and medium-sized farms that often welcome visitors and volunteers.

Start by seeing if any of them offer family walking tours, just to stack a little movement and outdoor time with information on what goes into growing your food. Many farms are eager for helpers around specific tasks and harvests;

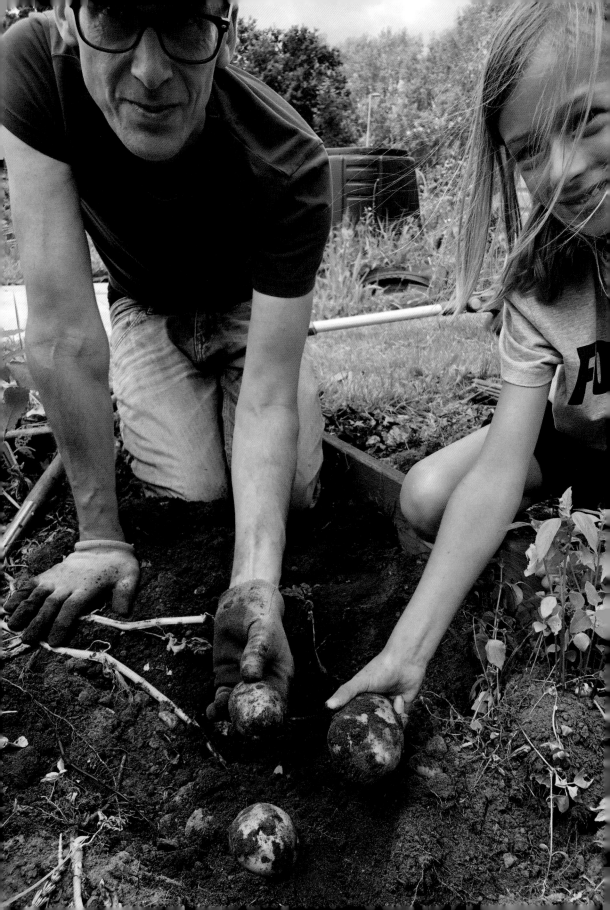

SHOW AND TELL

About two years ago we got an allotment at a community garden. Mainly it was a bit trendy at the time, although I did think it would just be fun to have a bit of space to try and grow things and learn on the job. I wasn't really thinking about the movement/nature thing at the time, but now I realize what a good MOVE that was.

We're a family of mum (fifty), dad (fifty-three), and a daughter (nine), and our garden simply gets us all out of the house, into nature, moving more, and moving the parts of our bodies we aren't used to moving. And boy at first did we all ache and moan about it! The digging, bending down, weeding, and preparing the plot alone was hard work for us, but seeing my daughter go from slouched in a chair, head down, playing on an iPad to digging with her hands in the earth for potatoes with sheer delight like she has found gold nuggets in the ground has been wonderfully worth it. And funnily, it is the odd-shaped ones she loves the finding the most, probably because you do not get those ones in the big supermarkets.

Even the smaller movements are worthy. On shelling broad beans she said, "Even though I know what is inside them, it is still so exciting doing it, running my fingers along the edge to break them open is so satisfying and relaxing." Hearing that made me relax too. In a time when we do worry about how our kids cope with everyday stresses, it just seems to prove to me that nature has the answers.

I have come to the conclusion that any crops we come home with are just a bonus. Being outside and getting that connection with nature is what counts.

—Lisa Thompson

there are mulching parties, potato digs, and strawberry-picking days, and if you can gather friends to join, you can stack your social and/or volunteering time with your food moves. Inquire about family work days too; what might seem like an unhelpful age can often just be a lack of exposure. Kids can learn to contribute faster than we think.

We have local farmers here who throw weeding parties, where they provide lunch and a green space for the kids to play in their group while we grownups catch up, talk about local issues, and just hang out, getting our nature time—all while weeding (because let's face it, there's *always* going to be weeding).

Look for U-picks where you can start gently and add movement to your jams and jellies (and P.S. if picking feels like too much, you can start by making jams and jellies!) and sign up for your local farm's newsletter so you're invited to official events, like those that teach about that farm's agriculture practice, demonstrate the care their animals require, or even let kids milk a cow or goat! Once you develop a relationship with your farmers, you might be able to contribute your family's moves to food more often!

HUNTING AND GATHERING MOVES

Traditionally, all kids are gatherers. Even kids that go on to be hunters start as gatherers. Gathering food is the foundation upon which children have always developed their knowledge and physicality. We think of "hunter-gathering" as an archaic, ancient practice with no relevance to our lives, but actually, kids are still natural gatherers, and gathering is still an easy way

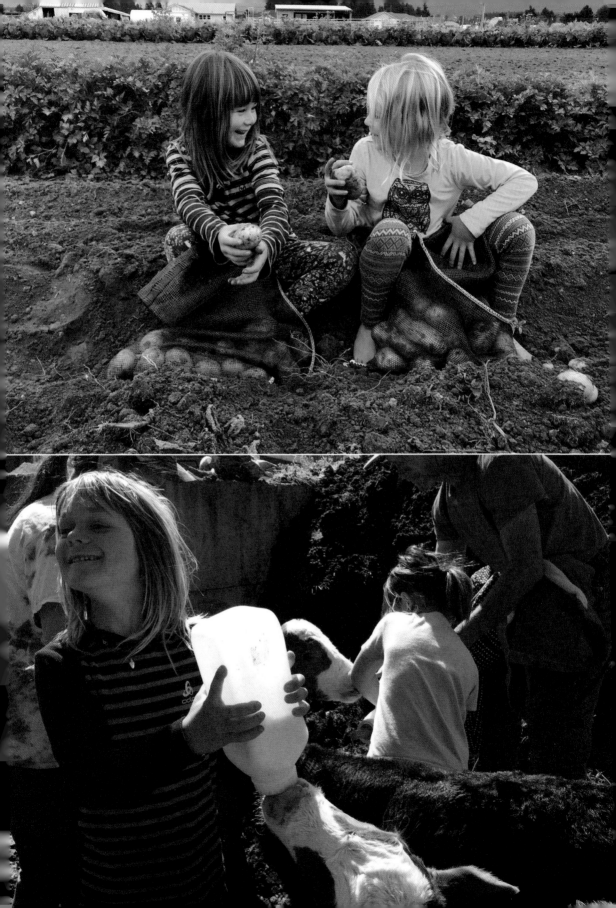

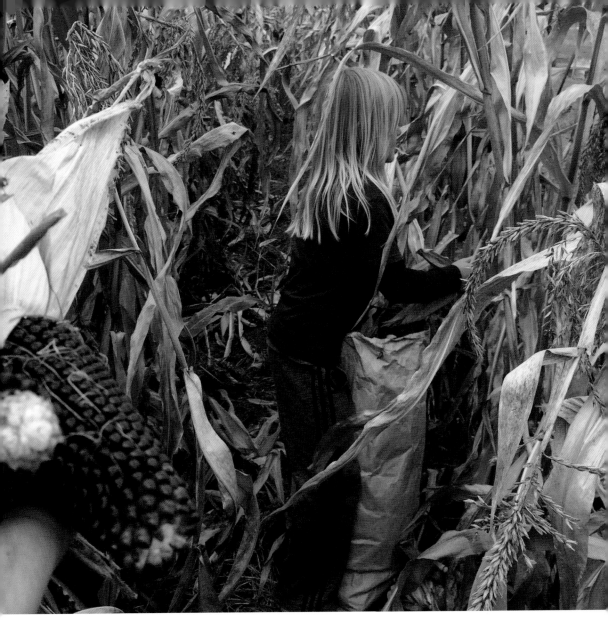

I've eaten thousands of pieces of popped corn in my life, but I'd never done any movements for that snack beyond the cooking and eating of it. But it turns out there's a local farm that grows popping corn, and our family was able to join in the harvest! It was a dynamic, glorious bit of time learning about the plant, filling and dragging heavy bags, being outside with each other and other animals, playing, and just hanging out. BONUS STACK: We made tamales afterward using the discarded husks. Ask your local gardener's club if popping corn can be grown in your area and which seeds work best.

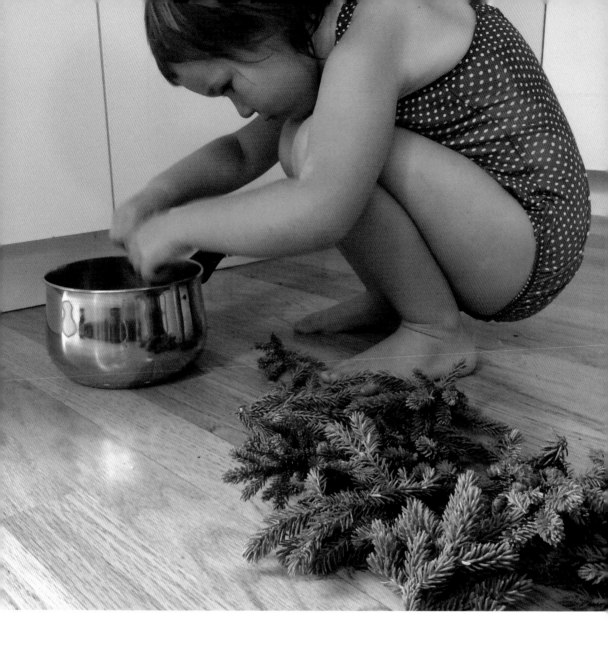

One of the simplest foods kids can start gathering is plant-parts for nature tea. Rosehips, dandelions, mint, wild chamomile flowers, spruce tips, rose petals— forest tea, or "Christmas tree tea," or whatever your kids will name it, is just a bit of nature steeped in hot water. Being able to use my harvest with almost no wait time? What magic is this?

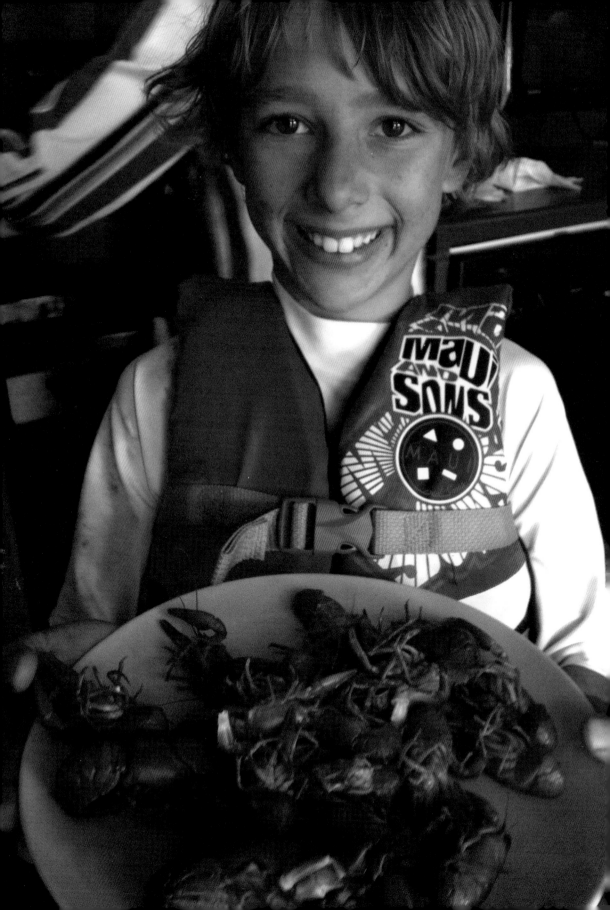

to find abundant nutrition. You don't need to be a wild plant specialist—you can find out which common weeds in your area are edible and start there. Dandelions, miner's lettuce, and wood sorrel are easily identified, early favorites that grow on lawns all over, and they're a perfect place for kids to start seeing the edible world around them. Berries are also an easy forage; depending on where you live, there can be wild strawberries, raspberries, blueberries, blackberries, cranberries, and more to be found even in cultivated urban parks, let alone what's available in wilder forest areas. Fruit trees are often within reach, especially if you have a climber on your hands. Gathering can be a part of your child's snacking when you walk, or part of a move-more mealtime mission: "Go pick some dandelions for the tacos!"

Hunting moves often require mentorship or teaching, so although hunting is a humanity-wide practice, some will not come by this opportunity easily. Still, hunting and fishing moves are out there to be learned. Fishing seems to be more available to more children—local fish hatcheries and parks often have a "kids fish" day. When kids go fishing they use a range of movement skills, from the "making movements" of fly-tying to the whole-body coordination needed for casting to the paddling and moving of boats. Other knowledge they'll need to absorb includes the ecologically responsible times to fish, which fish must be thrown back, and how to clean and cook their catch.

While hunting requires some of the most challenging moves, it's really just an aggregate of many nature-reading and playful nature moves kids can gather throughout childhood and adolescence: things like long-distance walking, games that have you moving quietly through a forest, identifying tracks and signs left by animals, using a bow and arrow or firearm, throwing and aiming, and knife skills that will help them process all animal parts (including hides—see "apparel-making moves") to avoid waste. Not everyone has access to or a desire to start hunting or fishing, and you don't have to—most movements and skills are easily practiced individually in a context that works for your family culture and landscape (for some fun nature-skills games, see page 318).

FOOD MOVES CAN BE ACTIVISM

While starting a patio garden or cooking more in your home might feel like quaint or luxurious activities reserved for those with extra time and money, it's important to know that many marginalized communities have identified the need for and are working toward food sovereignty—the ability to produce or gather their own food for independence from oppressive systems that keep them in a *food desert*: an urban area or other situation that grants no access to fresh or nutritious food. These are also often situations where folks are under-moved and under-natured, which ups the ante. Food moves are life-saving and culture-preserving for many people. Food moves are a form of activism that brings about social change. (For more information on what's going on in your area, search for and learn about Black, Indigenous, People of Color food movements online. Some of my favorite resources on these matters are *Farming While Black, The Color of Food,* and The Ron Finley Project.)

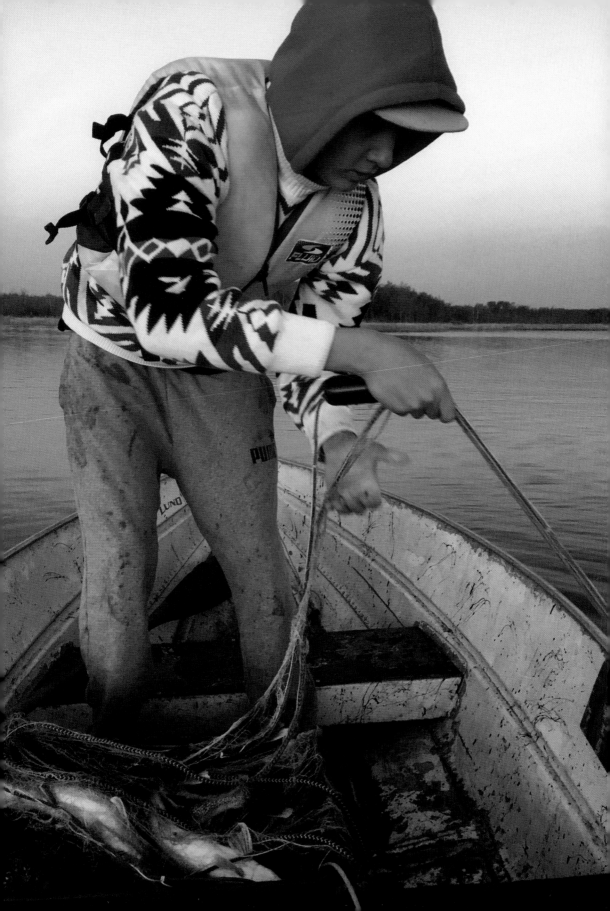

But wait! It gets even better! Food activism extends beyond addressing food deserts and sovereignty—we can also use *snacktion* as a type of ecoaction. How? Because every single food comes from the earth. Veggies? Obviously. Eggs? Yes, via chickens who eat foods from the earth. What about candy bars? Break down the ingredients list, and eventually you'll find yourself at some element provided by the earth. This goes for new synthetic meats, too—the laboratories and factories that make synthetic food are not only made out of the earth's resources, they are powered by those resources, as is the food being made there. Everything we eat takes something from the earth, which you probably already knew, but I wanted to say it anyway. Bear with me.

The exchange of movement for food was, initially, at the individual human level. You moved a lot to catch a fish, then you ate it. Through human ingenuity and a bit of chance when it comes to local materials, some societies created new food systems that required less of each individual's or group's movement, producing *more* food than before, and therefore they created conditions that could sustain more people.

Add in wheels, machinery, and irrigation systems, and over time we created larger and larger communities of more people able to eat food without contributing their own labor—which is great in the sense that it got us all here.

Flash forward a few hundred years and now the global food system has exploded in size. It's massive, with a lot of people eating and the food products travelling long distances, but there's not a lot of movement for the people or animals involved. It's a paradox. Food has never been moved so much at the industrial level and the people eating it have never moved so little.

The less we've moved for what we eat, the less we've moved altogether—because as I discussed earlier in the chapter, food is the environment in which our movement is most required. We've been shrinking our movement system, which means we require more food to be moved to reach us, meaning we're also expanding our food system.

Sometimes it's your local farmers moving for your food. That's easy to picture and easy to support. Do you know who's moving for the food in the grocery store, though? Do you know how the food was grown, and how the people growing it were treated, and how much they were paid? Do you know the ways fossil fuels were used to produce, transport, package, and again transport the food? Do you know if there were children laboring for your food? Do you know if they were even paid for their work?

This is not to get preachy. There are a lot of reasons we buy prepackaged foods that were industrially grown, and the main one is usually price. Big industrial operations are subsidized by the government and that means we can get that food cheaper, and you need to feed your family. I get it!

My message is, as usual, actually and action-y hopeful. Once you understand the inner workings of industrial food production, you understand that *every single food move* you reclaim—whether it's gathering, gardening, walking to the grocery store, or even just buying veggies whole instead of presliced—is a kind of activism. It's *snacktivism* (you're welcome). It's snacktivism for your own body, for your kids' bodies, for your community, for your planet.

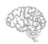 ## MOVEMENT BIAS CHECK-IN: FOOD

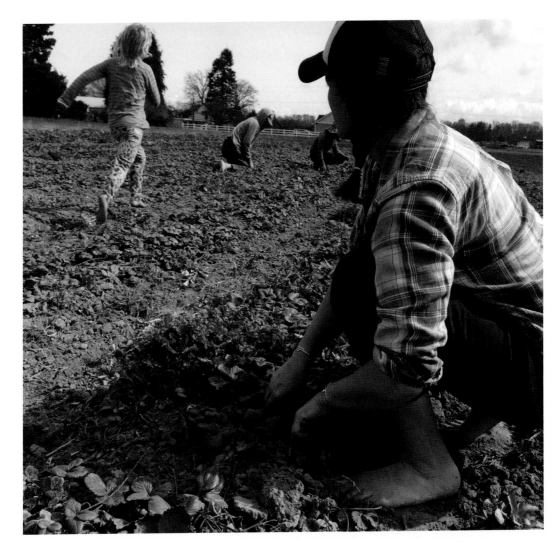

We all hold many beliefs around food, from which is the "right" furniture for eating and what counts as "good" or "bad" food, to the cleanliness of food and the value of working for our food.

Let's check in with our biases around food moves.

- Answer the question "Where does food come from?" Could you quickly outline the steps? How would children in your care answer? Hint: Ask them and see what they know about the food they eat.
- Do you think of or refer to food-related labor (cooking, harvesting, gathering, farming, gardening) as "unskilled"*? Do you think or refer to these jobs as "essential?" Do you talk to kids in your care about these jobs in a positive way? Do you mention food-jobs as a possible future career for them?
- What feels safer to you: eating items found in a grocery store, at a roadside vegetable stand, or in your backyard? Food you buy or food you make yourself? How does "wild food" make you feel? How do each of these scenarios make you feel?
- What are some differences between eating off a plate on the floor and eating off a plate on a high table?

*The term "unskilled" as we often use it has less to do with the required knowledge base (i.e., actual skill) and more to do with the fact that less formal education is required to do it, and thus it's work that people are paid less to do. There would be no humans without food producers, so it's pretty interesting to note (and ponder the effects of) labeling the people we depend on for our lives as "unskilled." We have created a scenario where we've placed little value on the knowledge and skills of food production, the most essential human work of all.

The challenge with widespread systems that need to be dismantled and rebuilt is that we are often trying to do this while still using them. As you and the next generation in your care learn to increase their food moves, we can decrease our reliance and theirs on an unwieldy food system that tends to exploit the planet's resources and other people's labor to benefit those of us not doing any food moves. Now, who's ready to take *snacktion*?

THE ECONOMICS OF SNACKTIVITIES

A favorite, twice-a-year snacktivity of ours is making salt. We load up the canoe, drive a few miles to the ocean, paddle out to gather Salish seawater and paddle back, load up the filled five-gallon buckets and the canoe into the truck, and then tend a five-hour fire, stirring, scraping, gathering, and then sifting and storing the salt. All in all, an entire weekend day is spent to, as a friend once said, "save ourselves the five bucks we'd have to pay for the salt at the store."

He can only see eight hours of work for five dollars' worth of salt, but I see the ecological benefits found in *traditional economy*—a perspective often missing when you've grow up in a culture with a *market-economy* point of view. By the end of that work, we had eight hours of time together, doing movements we don't get to do all the time (paddling, hauling, loading), and a five-hour fire that burned up our yard trimmings and warmed us late into the night. Our compensation was not only eight hours of outside time but a dose

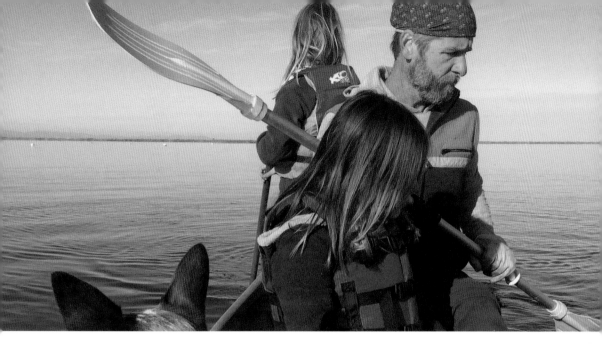

of *dark and magical* outside time. We all learned something new together. We had multiple hands-on science and knowledge lessons taught by the elements: how the salt water's salinity levels change with heat and evaporation, why in many places there's salt upon the earth, how minerals look different depending on their context, who are the people native to this area, how and what would they have eaten from the sea and what do they eat now, that the earth provides abundance and that an individual can exchange knowledge and movement for a portion of it. We took some personal responsibility for food we depend on for life and found a half a year's worth of salt—that we previously bought, imported from halfway around the world, produced under we-don't-know-what conditions—right in our own backyard. I do know where the salt is in the supermarket, but I have yet to find a way to meet *so many of our needs at once* on the shelves there.

One reason we might have a hard time moving away from industrialized food systems is because it's difficult to see beyond the in-hand product and

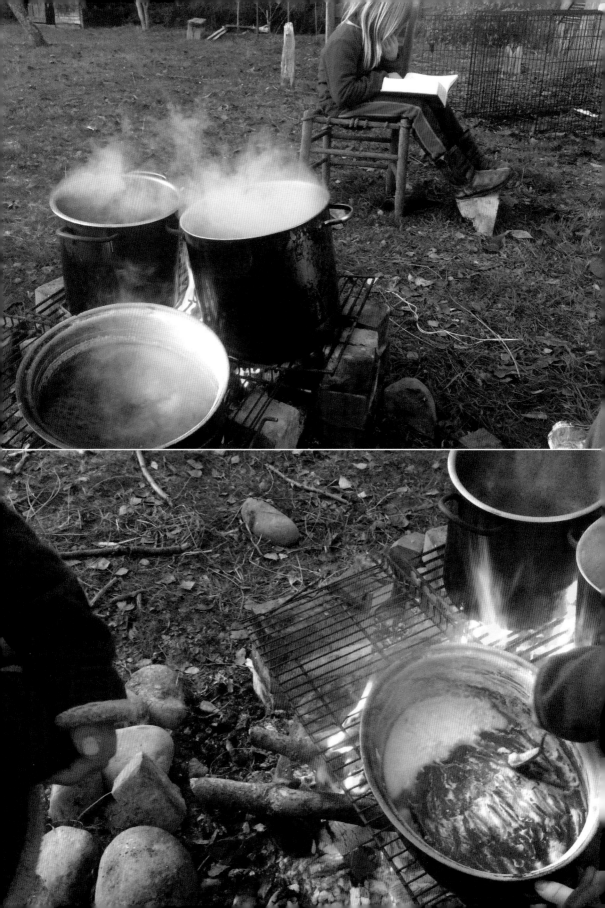

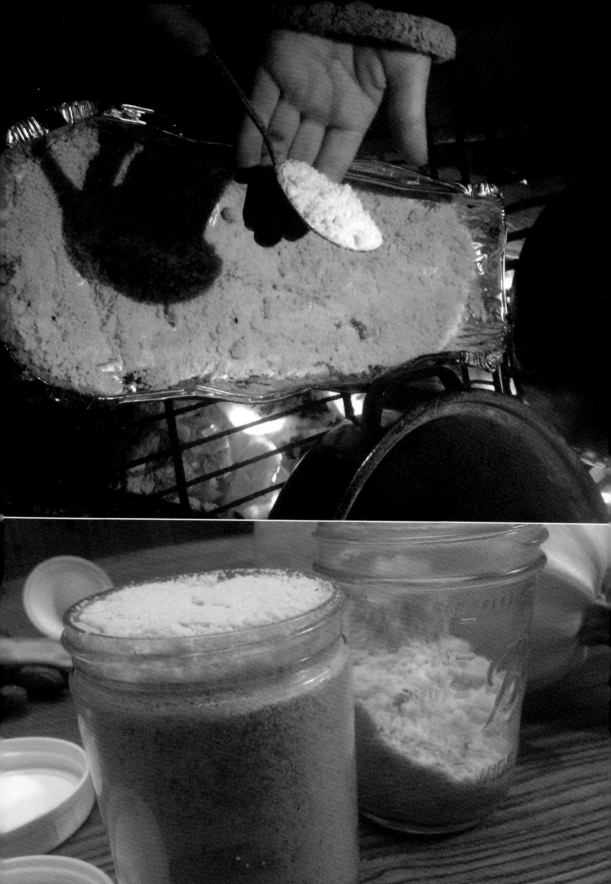

the out-of-pocket cost exchange. But our cost-benefit sheets are missing critical information. They don't reveal the deeper costs (other people, animals, the environment) or include all the true needs of humans and human children (see: the newly emerging "Vitamin Nature"). Our store-bought diets aren't providing all that food can. There are many nutrients to be found in making something we require, starting as close to the source as possible, and sharing this process and all those nutrients and knowledge with the kids in the community (salt-making party for the win!). These benefits are free though, so they won't show up on a label.

Snacktivities go way beyond food; they add *depth* to our calories. Kids get more time chatting with other kids and adults doing the food work; time to eat fresh berries and bend and squat and stretch in the sun; knowledge of plants, bugs, and birds and how they relate to the harvest; and how that all relates to the season. This is transmission of information over time. This is learning.

SNACKTIVITIES BY THE SEASON

Over the next few pages is a sample list of the year-round snacktivities where I live in the Pacific Northwest, which applies to many places in North America. I'm sure by now you're all in on the benefits of snacktivities. To recap: we're adding fun to food, AND ALSO increasing dietary nutrients, plant knowledge, food knowledge (including which peoples originally cultivated this plant, and when and where), responsibility, play, nature, and community.

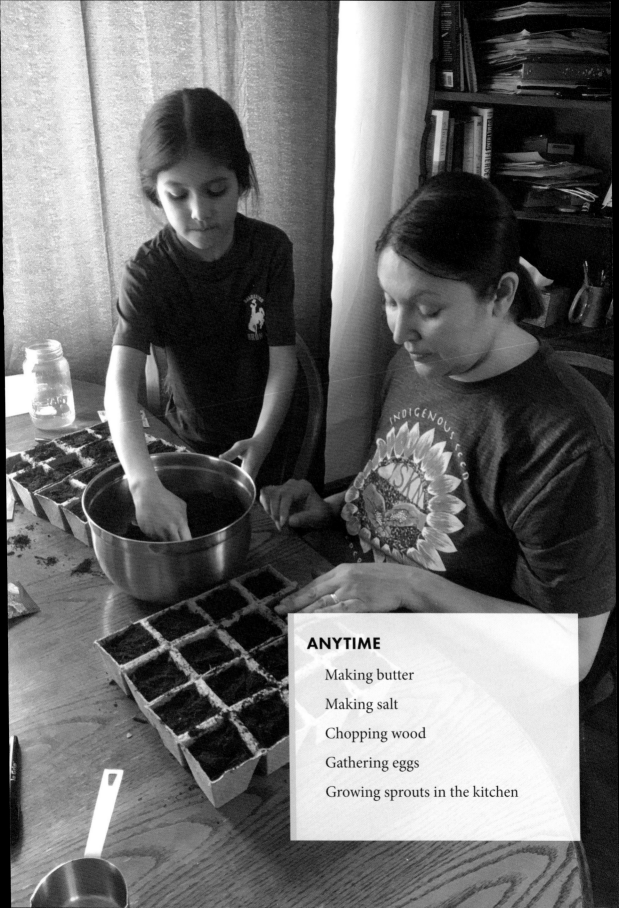

ANYTIME

Making butter

Making salt

Chopping wood

Gathering eggs

Growing sprouts in the kitchen

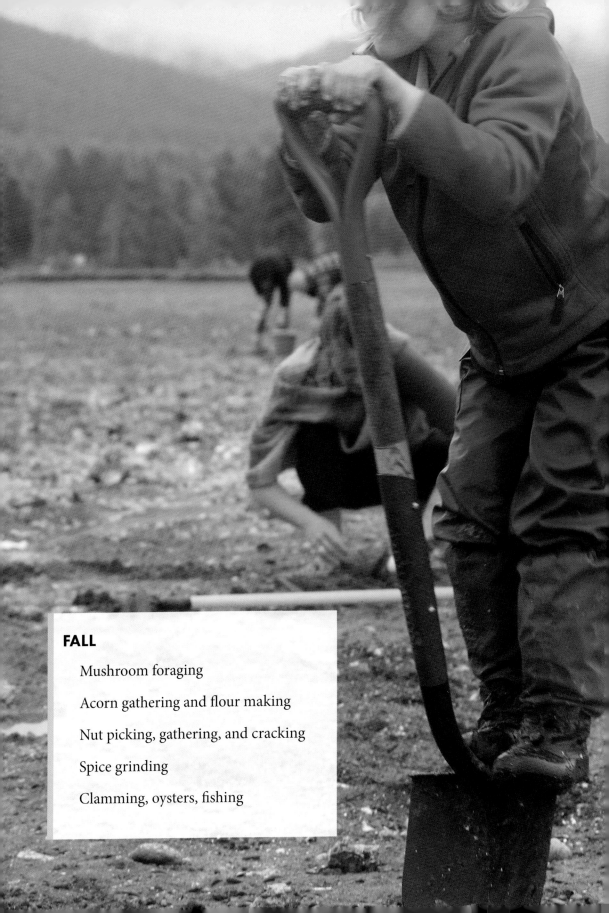

FALL

Mushroom foraging

Acorn gathering and flour making

Nut picking, gathering, and cracking

Spice grinding

Clamming, oysters, fishing

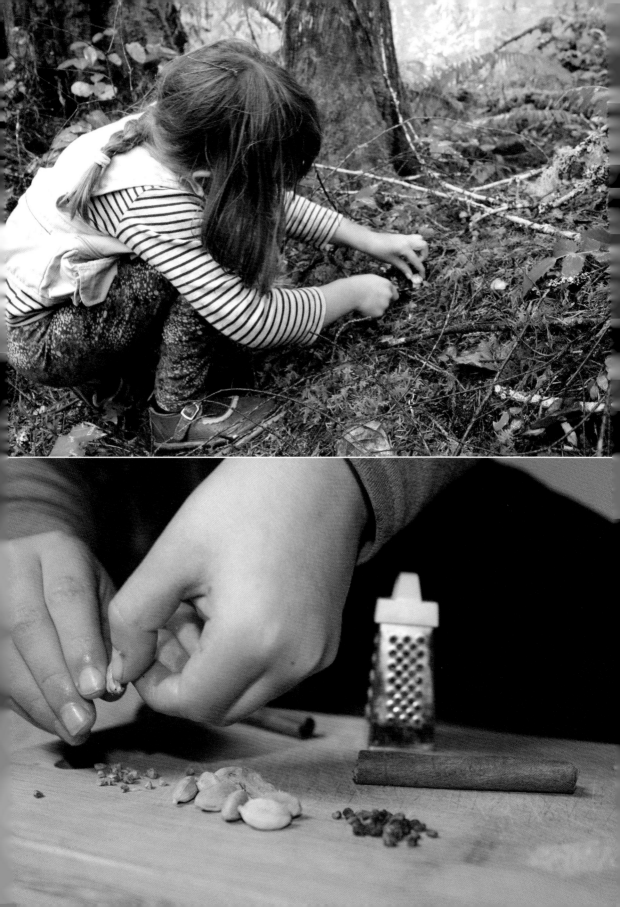

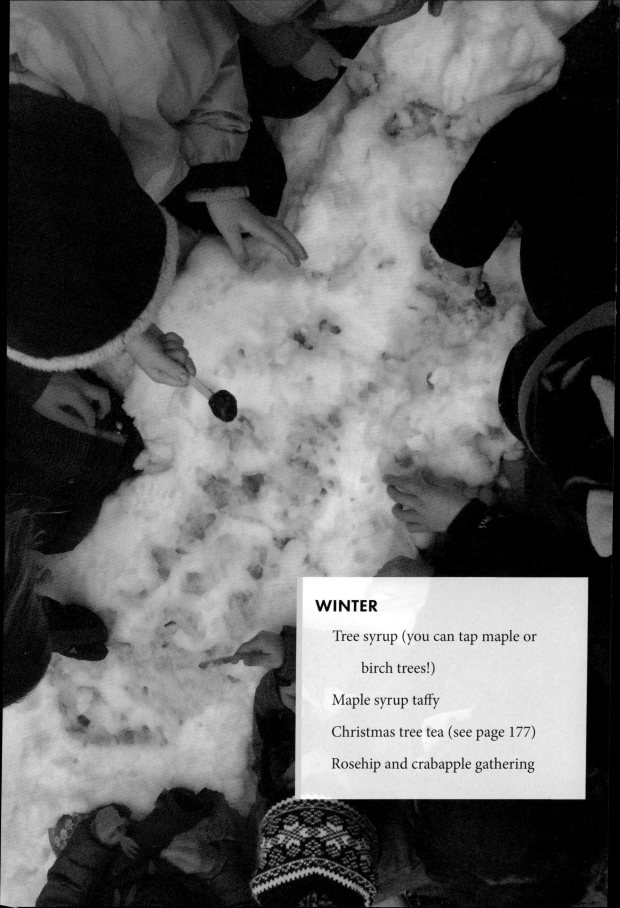

WINTER

Tree syrup (you can tap maple or
birch trees!)

Maple syrup taffy

Christmas tree tea (see page 177)

Rosehip and crabapple gathering

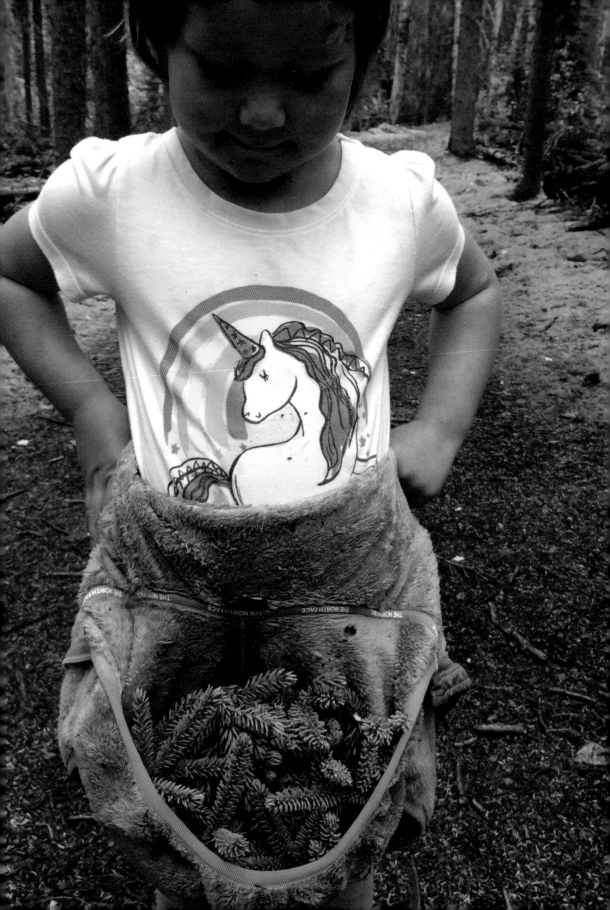

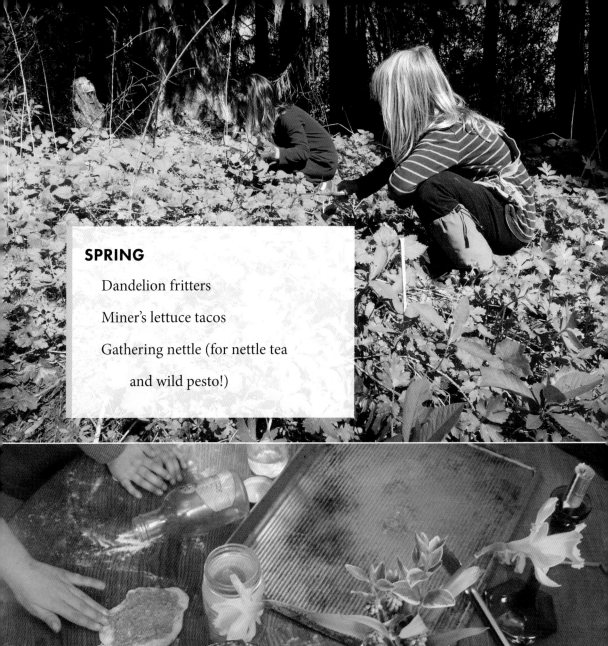

SPRING

Dandelion fritters

Miner's lettuce tacos

Gathering nettle (for nettle tea

and wild pesto!)

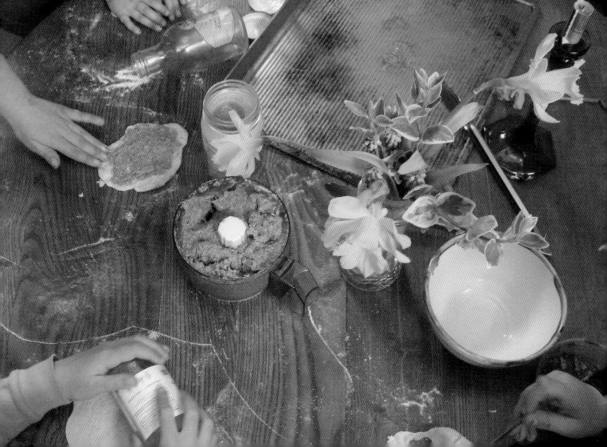

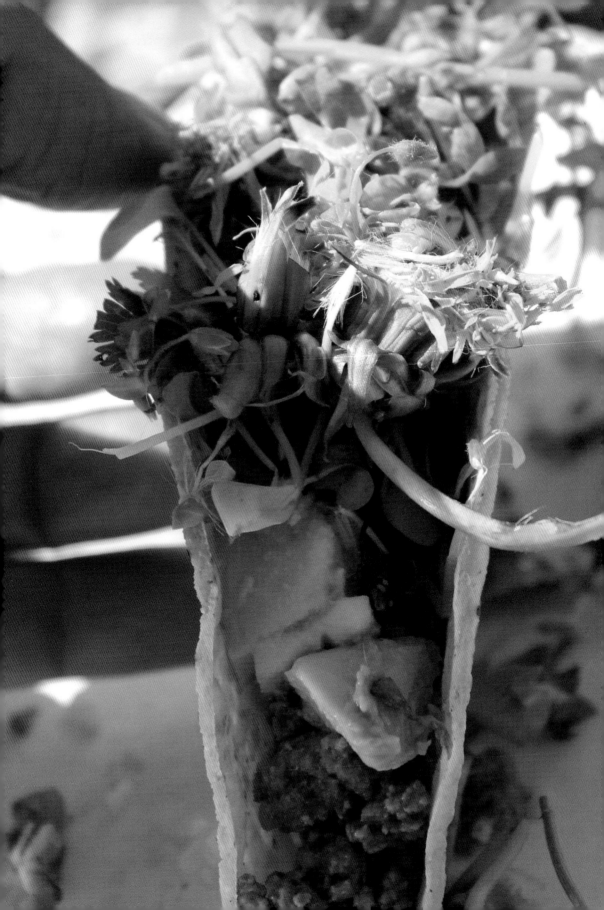

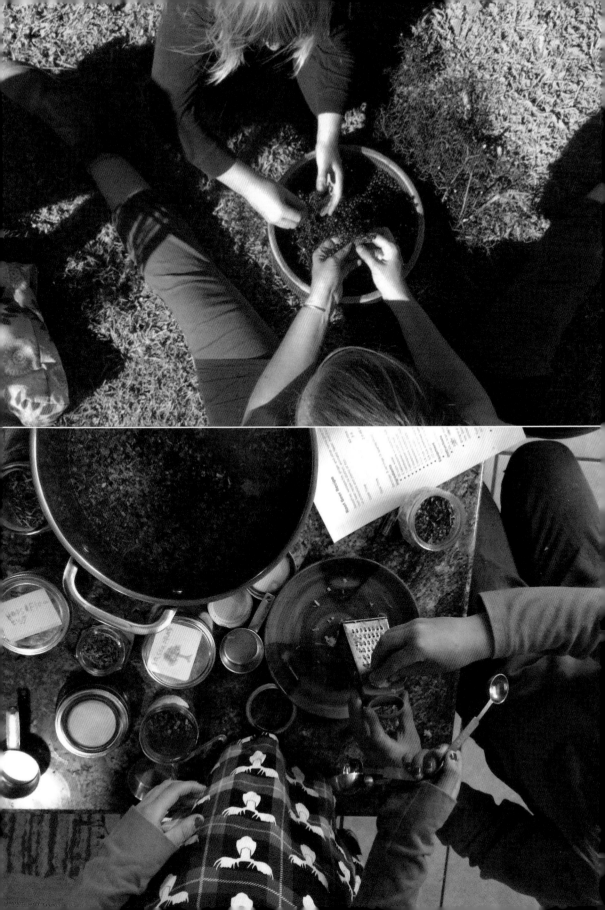

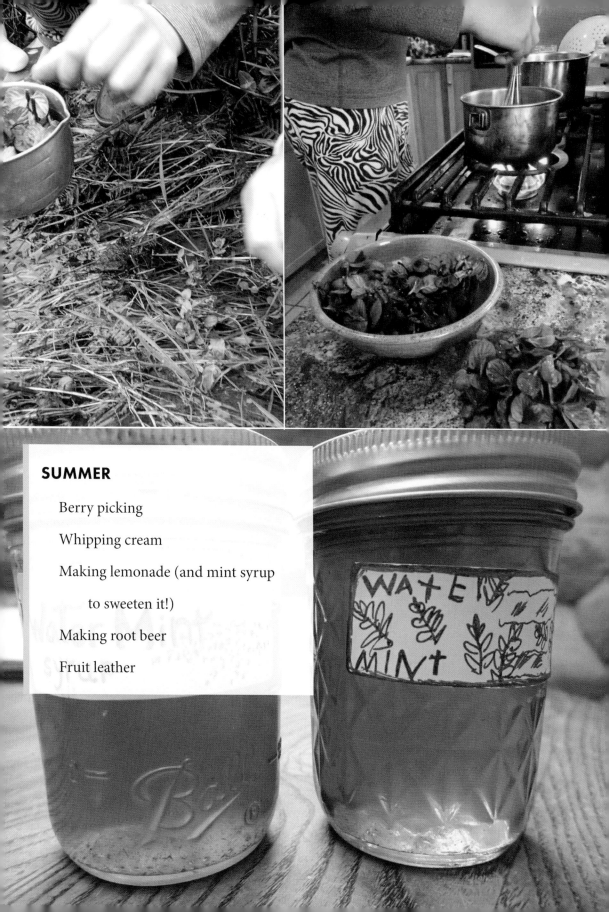

SUMMER

Berry picking

Whipping cream

Making lemonade (and mint syrup
   to sweeten it!)

Making root beer

Fruit leather

WATER
MINT

That's a packed snack, my friends. But you might be wondering where to start. (Hint: start with dandelions. Always dandelions.) The thing is, food moves have always been landscape-based, and every culture has local heritage snacktivities they might know about, even if they don't do them. If you're not sure, ask an elder in your area.

GO FORTH AND MOVE FOR FOOD

If the concept of snacktivities began with the idea of making food fun, I hope to deepen the idea. There's a relationship between humans, food, and movement that's been occurring since the beginning of human-time. To have lost awareness of this phenomenon is risky in itself, and there are also immediate consequences that affect our local and global community, as well as the globe itself.

Snacktivities—which start putting the movement, knowledge, and self-reliance back into our food system—hold the potential of restoring the movement that naturally occurs with a food and the responsibility of an individual's movement in the human food system. Food moves contain essential knowledge for our kids, about nature and the nature of where food comes from, as well as how they relate to the earthstuffs they require. Each day our kids wake up inside of our culture, get into their clothing, and eat. Food moves are essential, and a dynamic diet is not a luxury. Moving for the stuff you eat is a baseline human activity that many people are missing out on.

Movement doesn't grow on trees, and neither does nature education. Trees grow food, and it's because the food is up there that we are brought to movement and nature most efficiently.

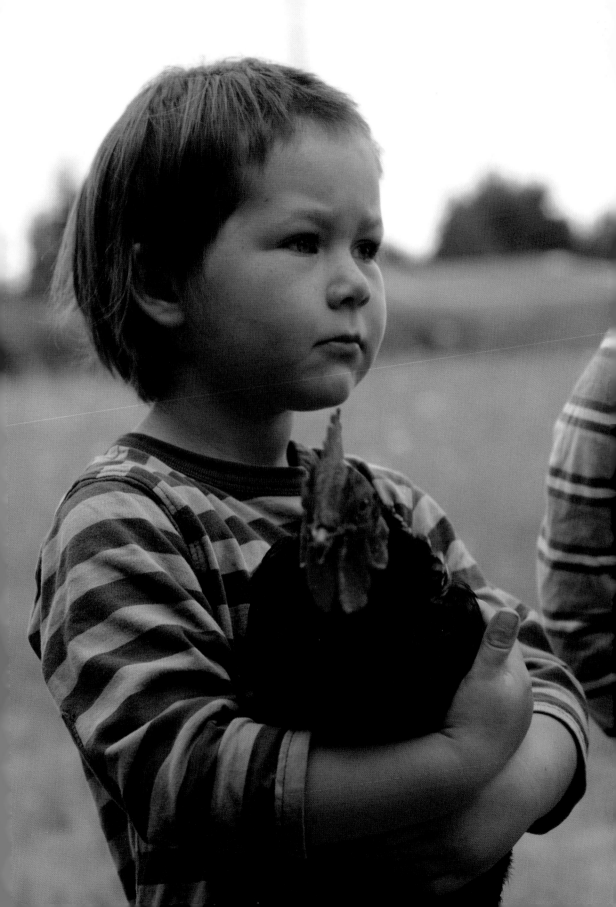

INDIGENOUS FOOD MOVES

Philip Brass is a member of the Peepeekisis First Nation in the Treaty Four Territory of Canada. He is a dedicated husband and father and a traditional knowledge carrier. He is a strong and emerging voice in the areas of Indigenous food sovereignty, land-based education, climate action, community health, natural movement, and traditional Indigenous knowledge and wisdom. Read more from Philip at philipbrass.com.

As a life-long hunter and fisherman within my ancestral home territory of what is now called east-central Saskatchewan, I'm grateful to be blessed with the physical ability and skills to live a life of walking, hunting, harvesting, and eating what remains of our traditional foods. I also enjoy the opportunity to share these often physically rigorous and yet incredibly rewarding spiritual lifeways with many school-aged children, youth, and adults. They are often starved for cultural identity, hungry for language, and often unknowingly hungry for movement and nutrition.

From infancy to death, Nehiyaw identities and rites of passage were based in roles and sacred responsibilities of a diverse and labour-intensive culture of food procurement. Nehiyaw babies were worn upon their mothers and grandmothers, as their feet were not to touch the earth outside of the tipi lodge until they reached two years of age. During these first two years of life, babies became familiar with the sights, sounds, and smells of the homefire, and the work of tanning hides, smoking meat, making clothes, and processing and using hundreds of medicinal foods and plant medicines. After a child reached the age of two, they would be acknowledged and

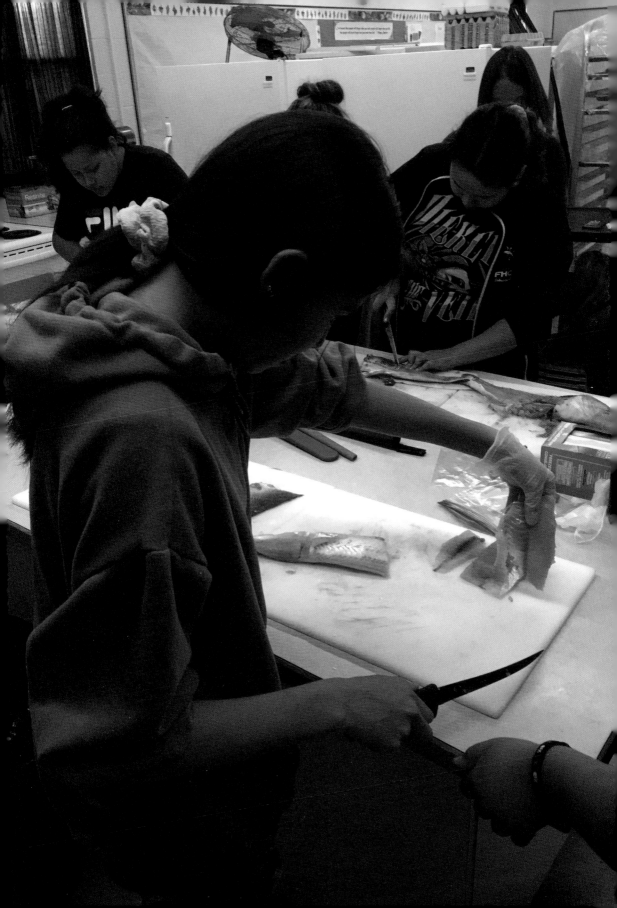

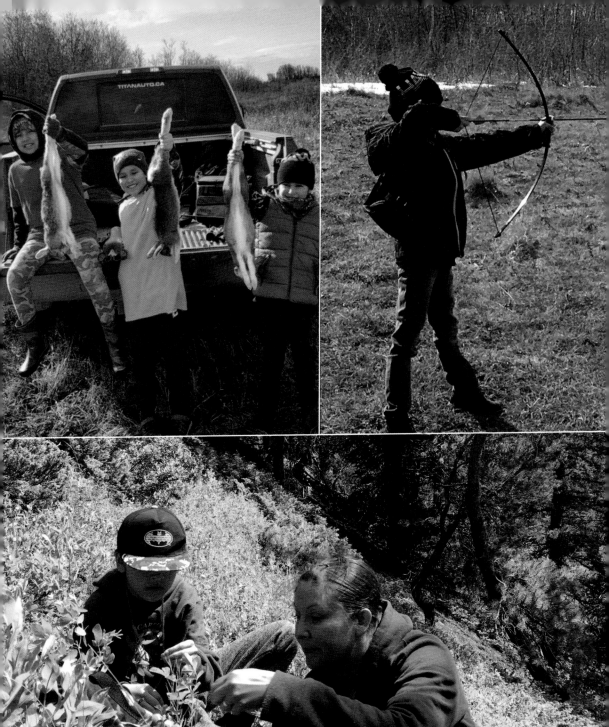
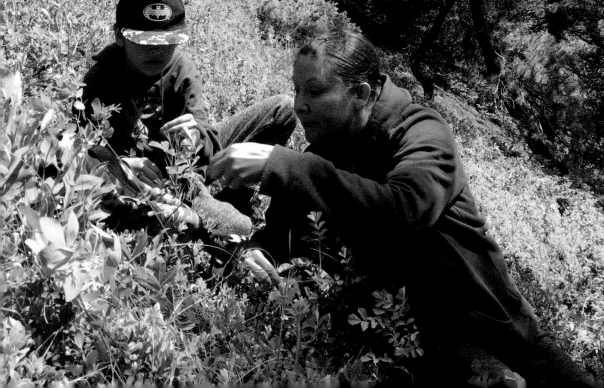

celebrated at an annual spring "walking out" ceremony, where they took their first independent steps upon the prairie grass outside of their home tipi lodge. At this time, the little ones would be gifted miniature food procurement tools to mimic the adolescent and adult lives they were to embark upon. The boys would receive little bows with arrows and the girls a miniature knife and pot, and the elders and various societies of the nation would give each child blessings for their life journeys ahead.

Buffalo hunting may have been the cornerstone of Nehiyaw life and food culture, but it certainly wasn't the only vital prairie food that shaped our bodies and seasonal movements. A rich variety of prairie plants, roots, nuts, berries, fish, and small and mid-sized game also led us upon an annual cycle of movement and harvesting over a span of hundreds of miles throughout the course of a year. From duck eggs to wild turnips, a rich life of movement, harvest, and trade guaranteed a life of alliances and renewal that not only benefited and served an anthropocentric purpose, but that of all prairie life beings, "all our relations."

My approach to parenting, one that focuses on cultural restoration, is not dynamic because we've called out movement as beneficial—the movement we wind up getting paddling, hiking, hunting, and fishing, is because our culture is inherently dynamic. To restore the culture is to benefit from the side effects of moving for our nutritional, communal, and spiritual needs.

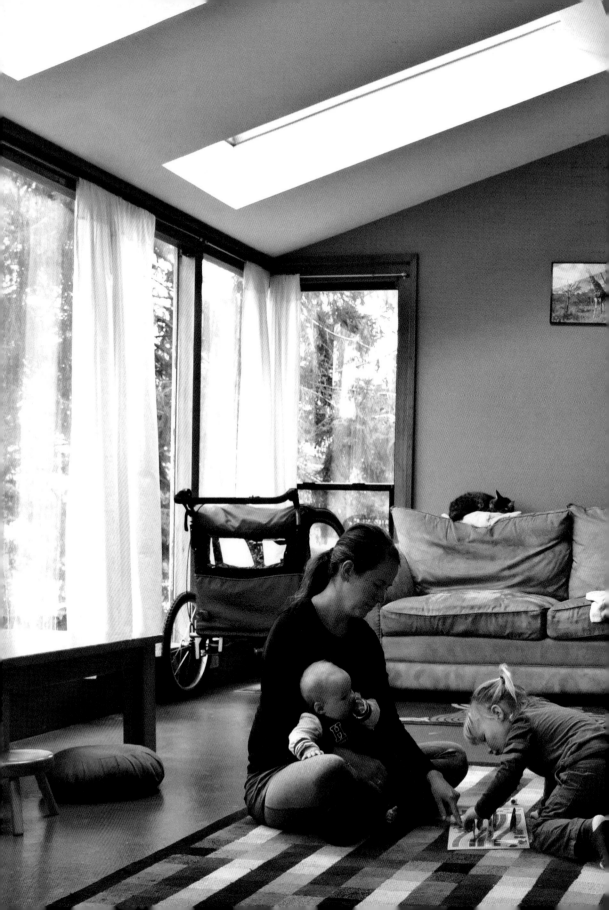

The Environment: Home

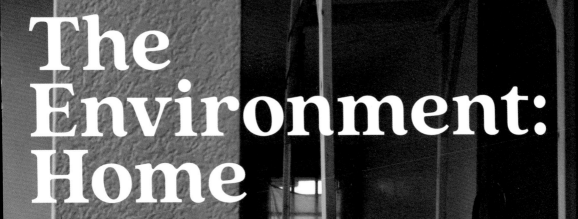

Our dwelling is a specified place for the indoor or sheltered parts of our lives.

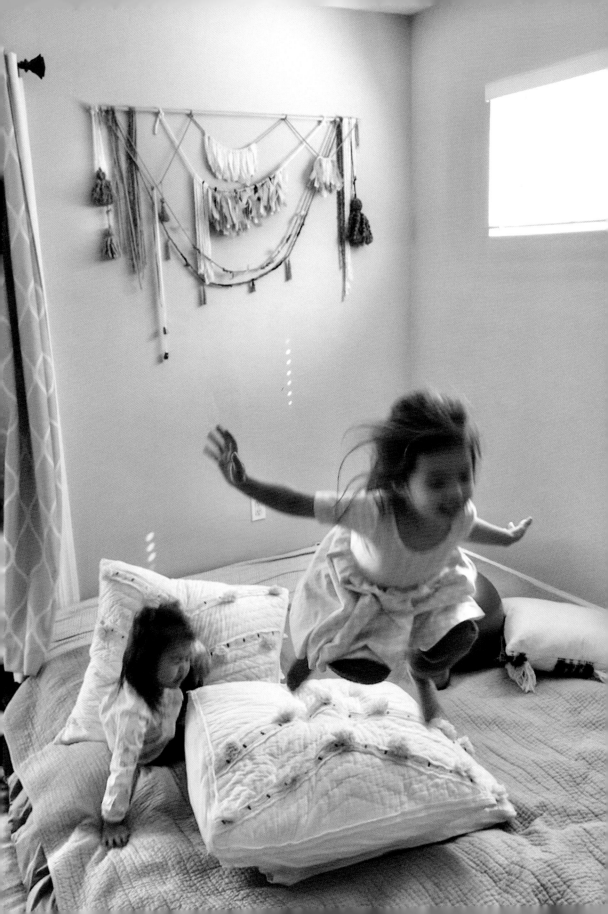

The Home Container

chapter five

O ur homes are like greenhouses.

Greenhouses are built to let certain elements in while keeping other elements out. Light and warmth? Yes! Cold and pests? Nope. What plant growers have discovered, though, is that while greenhouses are designed to allow some nutrients in, that same design has inadvertently blocked at least one: the movements plants need to thrive. As previously mentioned, a better understanding of plants' need for movement has led to greenhouses updating their practices (like hiring a team of "seedling strokers") to replace the plants' missing movement. Other growers, like my sprout-farmer neighbors, take that knowledge and simply supplement their sprouts' indoor time with a daily bout of outside "exercise" time. Really! They walk their flats of plants outside and back in each day so their infant plants become heartier. Whether growers use the more-movement-inside or the more-movement-outside approach, the plants' greenhouse experience has been improved—and human bodies overseeing plant raising got more movement too.

Human dwellings, like greenhouses, are designed to offer protection against the environment. Homes range in shapes and sizes, but the basic idea is the same across the board: to hold heat when it's cold and to stay cool when it's hot. They keep out wind, rain, hail, and snow, as well as predators like bears or mosquitos. Many animals make homes, too, which are always an attempt at controlling the environment to the animal's benefit.

The history of human shelters is likely as old as humans, but while the genes of anatomically modern humans have remained largely the same, our houses have evolved quite a bit. Just as human footwear has grown from simple foot coverings crafted from local food scraps (animal hides) to thick, stiff shoes made of rubber and plastic mass-produced in factories, homes have evolved from small mud huts to complex feats of building and material engineering, such as skyscraping apartments made of steel and cement.

Just as greenhouses don't facilitate any movement of plants and conventional shoes have inadvertently wound up blocking out kids' foot movement, our increasingly complex houses have been keeping growing kids from the nature and movement they need. Walls literally block out the non-human parts of the world (and thus the movement our parts would otherwise get as they passed through it), but more importantly, the new shape of our houses and the stuff inside them has reversed the way we use shelter. Instead of using inside as a place to rest after a day spent outside, we now spend most of our time inside. Our work, leisure, and community have all mostly shifted inside. Outside is now a place to pass through on our way to the next inside part of our lives. "Outside" is thought of as a *vitamin dose of nature*, used to supplement a *mostly indoor diet*. That indoor diet has been cemented by the fact that we have not only gotten rid of outside, but we've put all the things kids and adults use inside. This eliminates the pressures that once got us all to leave the hut naturally.

OUR HOUSES ARE MOVING US

Humans are tinkerers who have learned to shape their homes to their liking, whether they be made of mud or steel. There's a less-understood side of that coin, though: our homes are shaping us right back.

Just as tight or stiff clothing or shoes create cast-like physical barriers to movement by holding our bodies in place, the walls, screens, seats, and surfaces of our home promote certain repetitive body shapes. But the solution can be simple. There are ways to enrich kids' home life with movement and nature, and none of them require moving to a new place. You can facilitate more inside movement by bringing more "outside elements" inside, and bring kids to the outside parts of your home more often by bringing more "inside things" outside.

MORE MOVEMENT INSIDE

Human bodies are always being pushed and pulled by something. Even when kids are sitting "still," that in-place position moves the body in a specific way. Slouching in a kitchen chair moves the body differently than sitting upright in the chair does; lounging on the couch or squatting on the floor are both ways to take rest and be still, yet each is a unique movement shaping the body.

The skeletons of babies and children are not simply tinier versions of an adult's; their skeletons include much more cartilage than adult skeletons do. This cartilage is where bone growth—changes in length, thickness, and shape—occurs over time. This is also what makes kid skeletons more responsive to mechanical input than adult skeletons. Young skeletons adapt rapidly to the mechanical environment they're experiencing. While human skeletons continue to grow slightly and even change shape over a lifetime, their shape is set during the younger years and persists into adulthood. During childhood, bodies are like wet clay being molded to a shape that will be cemented in place. Younger bodies are constantly setting the stage for their future adult movement capabilities by how (and how much) they move.

Like trees, our genes contain the program for the *general* shape of each bone, but also like trees, the way we move creates the *nuance* of that shape. We can't move our thighbones in a way that causes them to look unrecognizable (a skeleton's thighbone is always clearly a thighbone), but thighbone movement during childhood affects the angle of their adult shape—an angle that makes the thigh better or worse at doing the movements required at the hip joint for standing, walking, jumping, etc.

STILLNESS LIKE NEVER BEFORE

Today's kids, *including infants*, are experiencing new-to-human-body environments: an unprecedented amount of indoor time, an unprecedented amount of "still" time, and an unprecedented amount of time being still *in one particular position*. Children have always needed to take rest, but never before have children taken so much rest in the positions they do today—curved into bucket seats, riding in cars, sitting in chairs, sitting at desks, lounging on couches.

The resting positions kids truly need have been used for many thousands of years, and these positions still help form the healthiest human shape. They include sitting on the ground in a variety of positions, squatting, and floor-sleeping. This is the "sitting playground" the body is most used to: a lot of different body shapes (kneeling, squatting, cross-legged, legs out straight) upon an ever-changing surface—flat, sloping, bumpy, wet, rocky, sandy, mossy, etc. In contrast, the indoor resting playground of today is repetitive. One body position (sitting), and one surface (cushioned). BODY BORING!

FURNITURE MOVES START EARLY

From an evolutionary perspective, the first "playground" for infants and their emerging shapes is the very low-tech practice of *being carried*. While being carried might seem like a passive activity (I'll just flop here while being carried, thanks!), babies sense what they must do to assist in the carrying action. Being carried is a dynamic and mechanically specific environment that gets a variety of baby body parts moving right off the bat.

Many human cultures have been transitioning away from exclusive baby-carrying for a long time, firstly using simple technologies that free up a carrier's arms, like a tied cloth for "wearing" a baby close. Uniquely, Western culture rapidly transitioned to a new environment: wheeled technologies that moved the baby off another's body. This effectively eliminated the carrying/being carried movement adults and infants produced as they moved from point A to point B.

Today, we're in an even newer environment: we're using baby carrying/holding technologies at a greater rate. More and more infants growing up in a Western culture are spending the majority of their time in a variety of "baby gear" that is often heavily researched for being safe for babies *during use*. But its effects on musculoskeletal development are rarely investigated or even thought about.

Simply put, our use of gear is shaping our children to the gear.

If a set of specific movements (the "being carried" playground) is part of the environment children's bodies are programmed to adapt to, and you

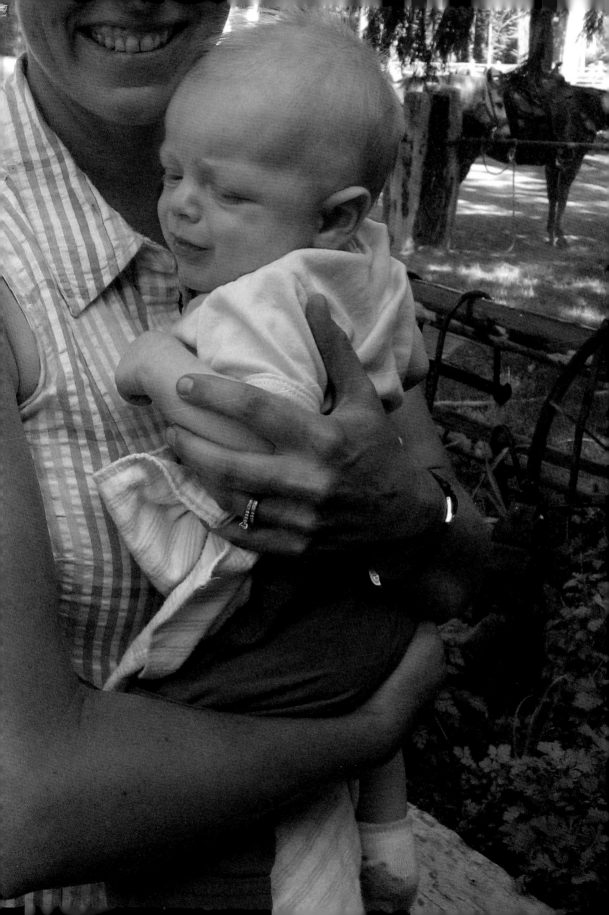

drastically change the playground (or eliminate it almost entirely, almost never traveling around with the baby in your arms), how does this new environment play out in the joints, bones, and other soft tissues of these infants once they grow up? This is what biomechanists and physical therapists are now starting to research and beginning to understand: how do "daily body positioning environments" affect the development of the musculoskeletal system, and how does this shape, coaxed out in the first couple of years, relate to adult ailments, including hip and knee joint diseases? Why might babies require periods of time with their legs working in a spread wide position, as found in some in-arm holding positions?

P.S. While baby-holding is good for the hips and other mechanical parts of the baby, *it is also good for baby in the broadest sense*. Babies are born with expectations of being held and carried as much as possible—this need is deep in their DNA. Also preprogrammed into a baby is its ability to send intense, passionate messages that something is wrong for them when it doesn't happen enough. In spite of what many parenting books advise, it might be worth seriously considering that this advice is based on only the needs we've identified so far (infant and child movement and its impact has *barely* been considered), and that a baby comes knowing something we don't. They really, really do need to be held and carried.

Carrying babies, like breastfeeding, creates infant movements that are becoming harder and harder to facilitate because of how our society is structured. It feels too hard to add more movement, especially because babies come without a baby-holding village replete with adoring older children and grandparent figures vying for cuddles (see chapter nine for more on all-important alloparents!).

But another angle available to most of us is recognizing that baby holding and carrying is an efficient way for everyone involved to move more. In fact, pediatric biomechanist Safeer Siddicky and his colleagues go so far as to note in one paper (see this chapter's references) that because of the robust, necessary movements it creates, we can think of upright baby-carrying (and a decrease in non-essential use of reclining baby-containers) as something with "public health potential."

Lately there seems to be a better understanding of how the health of one person affects and interacts with the health of people around us. Perhaps by framing the movement needs of a child as something beneficial to all of us, we can shift our culture in ways that will restore the practice of baby-carrying. That, or we'll invent baby-holding robots.

When it comes to their "movement diet," kids are overdosing on repetitive undemanding positioning and underdosing on any other movement nutrient from a very early age. This trend progresses right on through their lifetime. We start off in "baby-holding" gear and we transition seamlessly to kid- then adult-holding gear: all the chairs.

Sitting movements have become prevalent in all environments. But remember, we can modify our homes more readily than we can other places. Look around and try to figure out the body shape your home is creating most often.

STUDY SESSION: ARE DIAPERS APPAREL OR FURNITURE?

Whether you put them in the apparel or furniture category, diapers are an environment upon which children "sit" a lot; they're a bit of gear that affects the amount and direction a child moves their limbs.

Conventional, bulky diapers worn almost every minute of the day are a recent technology—less than a couple of hundred years old. And disposable diapers? Those have only been around since the 1950s. So what did parents do before? They used a method now called Elimination Communication (EC). Children, like adults, do not relieve themselves randomly; their toileting needs are predictable. Just as you likely use the toilet upon waking and after meals, children adhere to a similar timeline set by their physiology. EC is a process by which a caregiver quickly learns the "I need to go to the bathroom" signals (just like parents learn baby's communications for "hungry" and "tired"), brings them to a certain body position over a toilet or bowl, and as I learned, makes a sound when the baby eliminates (we used a sound like snake hiss, "sssssssssssssss"; other families we know used a low whistle).

The baby learns that the sound, body position, and toileting action go together and learns to eliminate when the caretaker creates this environment. EC has been used for millennia and is still used in many parts of the world today where resources and manufacturing are limited.

Diapers are undeniably convenient, but they're also a new environment. Along with their tremendous expense and waste (there are millions of tons of diaper garbage created in the U.S. alone each year, and cloth diapers also use up a lot of water and electricity for washing and drying) as well as issues associated with poor use practices (rashes and infections), diapers change how children move.

Just as researchers are tuning in to how baby gear like baby carriers and bottles affect developing anatomy—in order to better understand the situation as well as to improve the technologies—there are now efforts to learn how diapers affect infant and child movement. A study of spontaneous movement in three-month-old babies wearing a variety of diaper shapes while lying on their backs showed that the legs of diaper-wearers moved more slowly and with less range of motion; naked babies moved their legs more freely. Studies of thirteen-month-old and nineteen-month-old walkers showed more falls and missteps in diaper-wearing early walkers as well as wider, more immature steps. Diapers are a brand new playground in which the rides all force your legs apart, just a little bit, all of the time. Annoying, right?

EC is the best solution my family came up with, even if we couldn't do it all the time. It's free and doesn't create any garbage, but it's not always practical. For financial and other reasons, many parents aren't with their kids all day, every day throughout the first two years. Caregivers must also be able and willing to communicate with infants in this way.

We must be free to choose our path when it comes to dealing with children's toileting, but many parents have not been presented with all the available options, especially one—EC—to which children are well-suited. While it might not always be practical, EC is pretty simple. The way we approached it was to cultivate the practice right away and then use it when it was most practical for us, in an EC-diaper hybrid.

No matter the toileting environment you create, it's easy to give babies time to move without gear or clothing binding their waists or thrusting their legs apart by simply adding pants-free time. Too cold? They can go diaper-free in thin pants. If you have an emerging walker, give them some diaper-free walking time. This is where EC comes in handy. We might be keeping kids' hindquarters under wraps because we're worried about messes in the home environment. If you and your little one have invested time in learning how to communicate about toileting, you'll know when they need to be brought to a toilet to avoid the floor puddles...and they'll know they're being received. P.S. Stacking diaper-free walking time with a little outdoor time is also an option, weather permitting!

We're often trapped by the idea that doing something partially doesn't count. But isn't it good to eat some nourishing meals, even if not all of them are? Isn't forgoing plastic water bottles some or most of the time better than never? EC does not need to be used exclusively; cultivating this reflex early on and using it some of the time can pay off when it comes to kids getting more of the movements they need.

Bender, J.M., and R.C. She. "Elimination Communication: Diaper-Free in America." *Pediatrics*, June 21, 2017.

Cole, W.G., J.M. Lingeman, and K.E. Adolph. "Go Naked: Diapers Affect Infant Walking." *Developmental Science*, September 7, 2012.

Gima, H., M. Teshima, E. Tagami , T. Sato, and H. Ohta. "The Shape of Disposable Diaper Affects Spontaneous Movements of Lower Limbs in Young Infants." *Scientific Reports*, November 7, 2019.

BABY-CARRYING POSITIONING

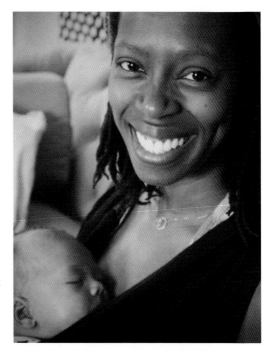

Dr. Tia Ukpe-Wallace is a physical therapist specializing in pelvic health and self-care through body literacy. She shares her perspective on baby positioning. Find more from her at selfcarephysio.com and at @selfcarephysio on Instagram.

As a physical therapist and a mom, I am a huge proponent of inward-facing baby-wearing. I wore my baby, who is now six years old, for the first six months of her life until she could start sitting up on her own. Not only was inward baby-wearing a hugely intimate bonding experience for me as a first-time mom, but I also knew that it would have great benefits for her overall hip development. Whether it is carrying baby in arms or in a baby carrier, I knew that her hips would be in the most optimal positioning, which would ultimately set her up for ease when it came to crawling and eventually walking. In addition, when I held her in my arms, she would also learn to use her leg and hip muscles for holding on to me as I held her in one arm and performed tasks with the other.

As I have seen her continue to grow and develop, my daughter continues to remain versatile in her movements and able to maintain good hip and leg strength and mobility, which I greatly attribute to optimal positioning as baby.

How many seats beckon a child? How often are children required to use chairs to access the stuff they need? We can look for easy ways to remove "standard chair movements" from places they're not truly necessary and change the sitting movements in the home environment. Let the chair-weaning begin!

STACK IT ON THE FLOOR

Take a moment to think of the height of the surfaces kids might use in a home. In the kitchen, what surfaces do they use for cooking or eating? What about their sleeping surface? Sitting surfaces? Homework surfaces?

Every surface's height affects the body shape of the person using it. The original surface for humans was the ground—a surface that occurs everywhere on land, and a surface that requires many body parts to move as it is being used. Moving to and from the ground using only our own body power is a fundamental human movement and is one of the reasons we have the anatomical shape we do. Yet many humans in our culture have lost the strength and mobility to do this in many parts and are simultaneously facing musculoskeletal diseases and injuries.

To figure out why adults might lose some of this body function, look at our modern greenhouse-like homes. We've created abundant features such as desks, tables, chairs, counters, and toilets that elevate our most-used surfaces from the ground. This makes life easier in the short term but harder in the long term. This is because it largely eliminates our immediate need—and eventually our ability—to move our hips, knees, and spines through their full range

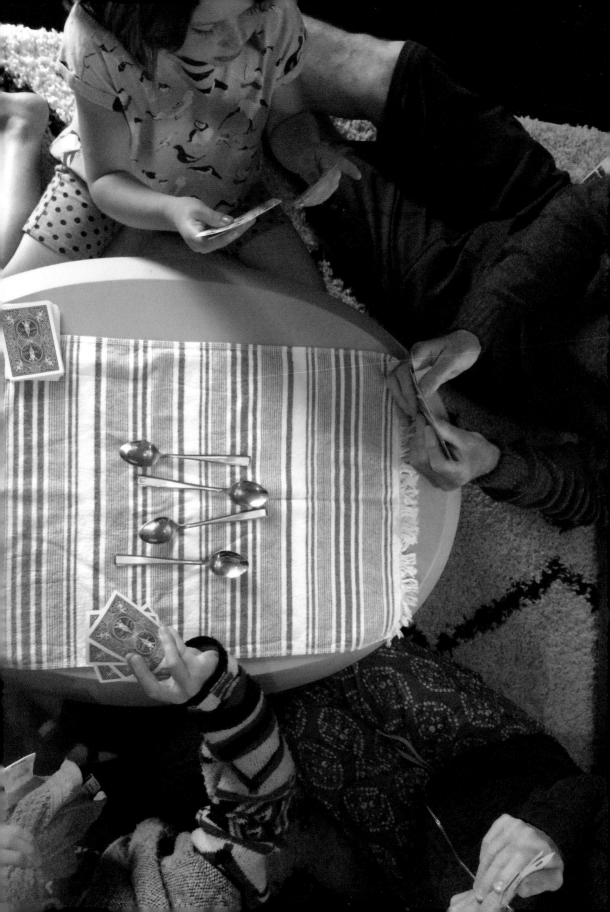

of motion. It is not a coincidence that the movement therapy adults are given for stiff ankles, knees, and hips includes exercises that articulate these body parts in the same way they'd have to move if one were getting to and from the ground! It is much easier to preserve movements from a young age than to reclaim them after they are lost, which is why dynamic kid environments pay off not only in the immediate sense, but in the long term too.

Adding leg movements doesn't require getting more stuff for your house; you can increase your kids' movement by taking stuff *out* (or at least out of the way). We need *less* furniture holding kids in the same positions and blocking their access to the most dynamic part of their home: the floor.

Stacking more movement, especially of the hips, knees, and torso, into home-time can be as simple as moving tasks you're already doing down to the floor. Reading, writing, art projects, entertainment time, family games, and even eating don't have to happen in the shapes we're accustomed to. These can be done entirely on the floor or at lower, coffee-table-height tables that make the use of a chair obsolete.

We've used a variety of already-low coffee tables—as desks, play tables, kitchen counters, and dining tables—and we've cut down the legs of taller tables too. We've also played around with the best height for eating, settling on 16 inches/40 cm tall for now. The height is often predetermined by the height of the furniture we're modifying, and we can adapt our bodies to that height via bolsters, stools, or cushions.

Even while they're staying still, kids can get different movement nutrients out of "just sitting there" by changing how and where they sit. An easy way to do this is allow kids to use existing furniture creatively. You can talk to kids about the movements you're not okay with (say, those you think might break your furniture) while giving permission for many more.

You can also swap conventional chairs for more dynamic pieces of furniture—like ottomans, poufs, cushions, and exercise balls—that offer many different versions of sitting, each with their own muscular use.

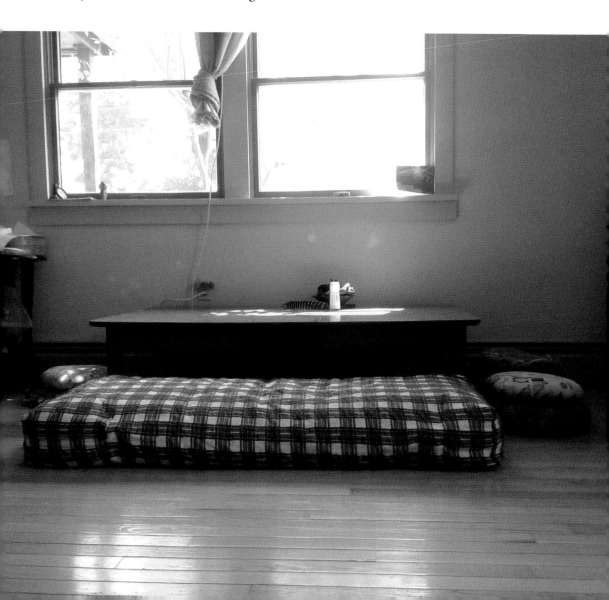

DON'T BLOCK THE SQUAT (OR OTHER FLOOR MOVEMENTS)

The ground surface facilitates many shapes, one of which is squatting. In general, human bodies come with squatting hardware and software. Squatting not only gets you to and from the ground, it's how many humans the world over take rest (and toilet). With the exception of those with certain disabilities, young children start off squatting. In cultures that continue to

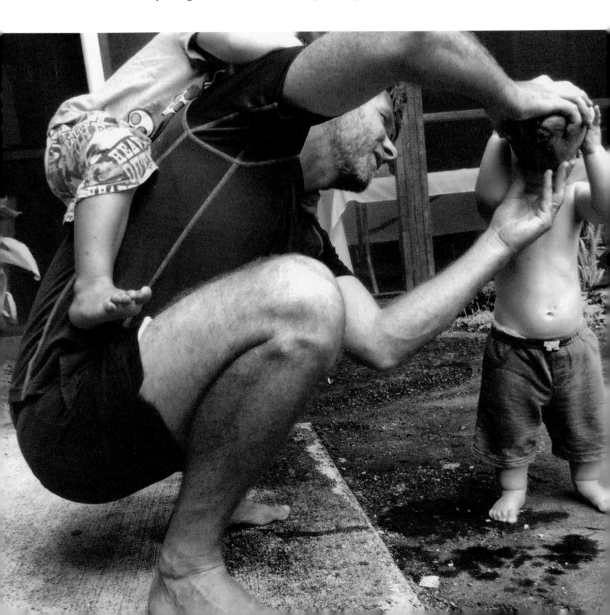

squat, this ability remains. In non-squatting cultures, where people are given seats instead and don't see people around them squatting, kids lose the ability to squat—and become adults who cannot. Is squatting valuable, even when you don't need the movement negotiating our environments? I say it is. The gifts of a squat go beyond the act of taking rest there. Additional values include maintaining a full range of motion in our hips, knees, and ankles; strong thighs, buttocks, and pelvic floor; the ability to get off the floor if you've fallen; the ability to reach and care for your feet.

It isn't clear yet whether a lost squat can ever be completely regained or whether some aspect of it is permanently lost (squatting as the skeleton is forming seems to retain flattenings called "squatting facets" in bones at the ankles). Regardless, although we rarely see them in Western society, squatting kids become squatting adults simply by regularly taking a squat instead of a seat. If they don't, it's hard work to ever get it back.

Squatting isn't the only floor movement kids can use. The joints in the body allow us numerous sitting positions—a few examples are cross-legged,

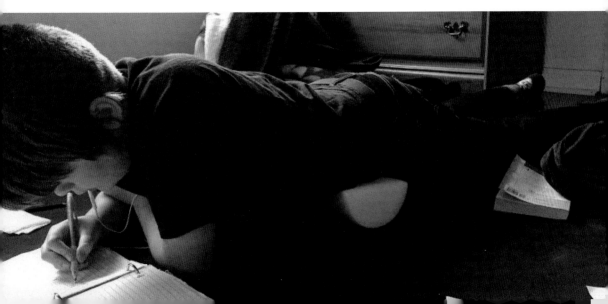

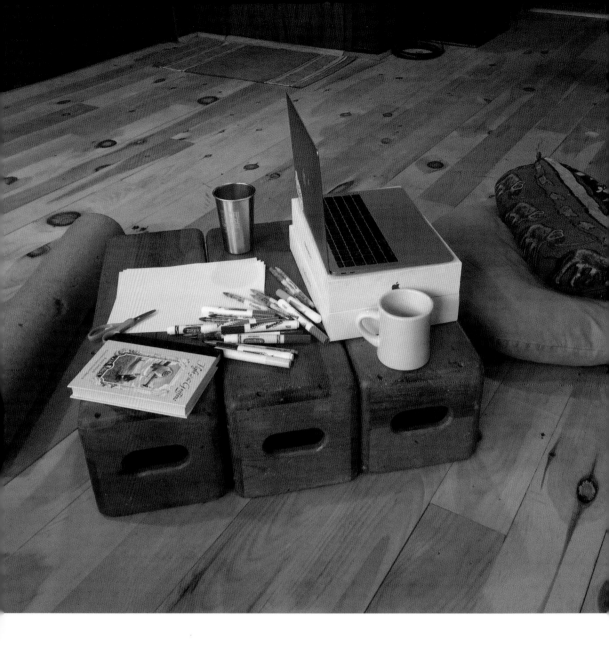

If kids are in one position for most of the school day, create a home-work station that offers them more movement. This can be created with items you already have at home, and you can opt for a setup that utilizes the floor or one that uses a standing position. Seats can include cushions or balls and other options that allow them to fidget while staying more or less in the same place.

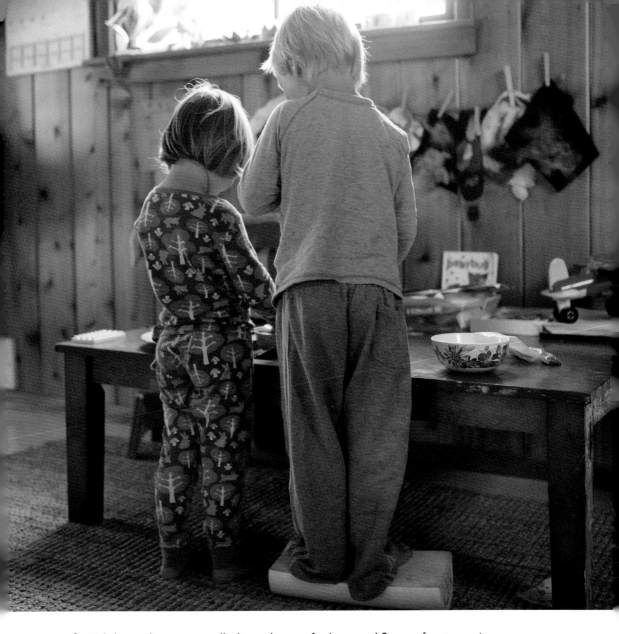

While my home actually has plenty of what qualifies as furniture, I use the shorthand "furniture-free" to describe the lack (or reduction) of padded, cushioned sitting-and-sleeping furniture many houses are full of. I started sharing photos of my furniture-free home on social media, and many others have shared how they have set up their spaces as well. Furniture-free homes can be beautiful, cozy, and even elegant—our need for adornment goes for our dwellings, too! You can see many examples of how folks have stacked their needs for shelter, adornment, and movement by searching #furniturefree.

legs folded to the right or left, legs straight out in front, or kneeling with one or both legs tucked beneath the sitter. Kids might even be more comfortable taking rest or doing their homework lying on their bellies. If you're concerned about their form, or if they note discomfort in their favorite resting position, offer up the idea of "good form" and how to bolster their body. For example, a small pillow or prop supporting the front of the pelvis if they're lying on their stomachs immediately decompresses a lower back. They're getting a break from chair-sitting in a body-beneficial way.

HANGING

The relationship between humans and trees goes deep. The movements necessary to use trees as a place to hide, shelter, or source food have literally formed our anatomy, including our ability to "monkey around" on our arms—a swinging movement called *brachiation*. The complex anatomy of human shoulders includes joint and tissue shapes that allow our arms to reach out in front of us, move overhead, and then sweep behind us as we hang on to something and swing beneath it.

If you think of baby shoulders as clumps of clay, and "outside" and "trees" as the environment that kid shoulders have inhabited the longest, then it's clearer how these parts depend on pulling and reaching movements to develop fully. These motions mold the hands, arms, shoulders, and torsos into structures that are able to move robustly in the future.

Human anatomy comes pre-stocked with the parts that allow us to hang from and move through overhead branches, but if they are to develop properly, this movement must be practiced as we form. It is the practice that sets the shape.

Our modern home environments barely move our arms, and with the increase in media time, kids' hands, arms, and shoulders are being molded in a way that makes it hard for them to use their arms for anything but swiping and typing. Average grip strength in 20–34-year-olds was less in the 2000s than it was in 1985. Researchers suspect the decline in physical labor as a cause (see the "grip strength" section in this chapter's references for details). But does that matter, given we've set up a culture where our movement is obsolete? If we can get everything we need with a swipe, then shouldn't we just make sure our kids are *really good at swiping* to ensure their success? Why

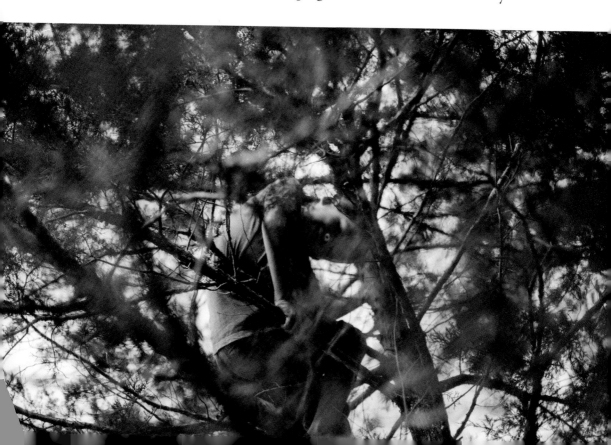

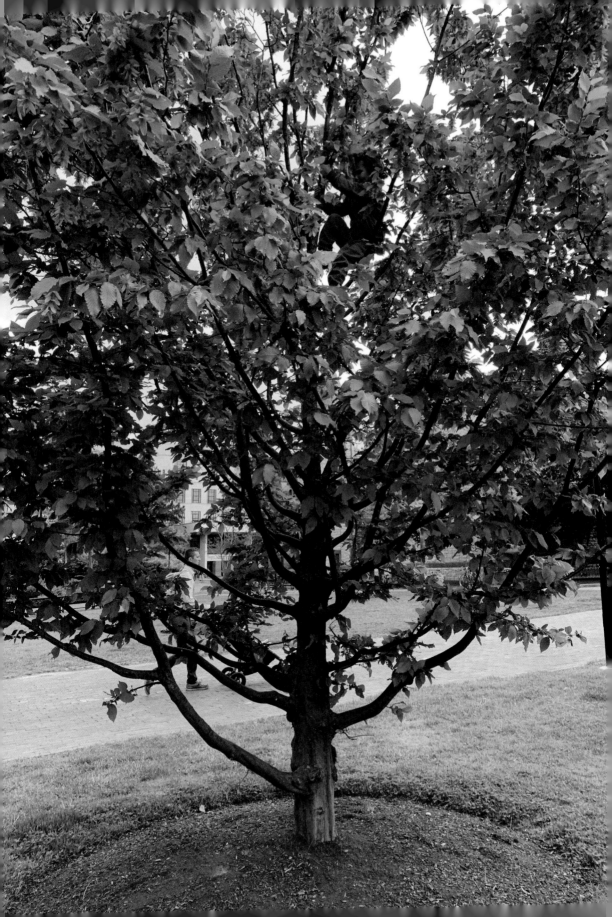

bother with archaic movements like squatting and hanging and climbing and walking when modern environments don't require them?

That argument is logical, but it misses some deeper issues. Body movement does more than shape and strengthen our bones and muscles. Not only do we humans depend on our body strength to take care of us in more threatening circumstances, but also movement, in real time, works with the heart to help circulate blood. Lungs depend on musculoskeletal movement and the musculoskeletal system's strength to get enough oxygen. The way kids' bodies are able to use the energy from food depends on movement, and kids' brains function better in a body getting enough movement. It used to be that the environment demanded our movement AND our body needed it; now just our body needs it.

What does this have to do with hands? First, research shows that adults and children with low grip strength experience poorer health. Why is this? It's not clear, but from a biomechanist's perspective I suggest that it's an indicator that at least half of the body is severely undermoved. Not only are kids (and adults) barely moving to our capacities, when we *are* moving it's almost always the lower half of the body. Relatively speaking, our upper bodies are less functional than our lower bodies due to our environments. Even in those getting more movement, the movements we choose rarely involve the upper body. This is a particular problem because the lever-and-pulley system of the upper body—the way the bones and muscles connect there—indicates that muscular strength in the arms, chest, and upper back directly impacts

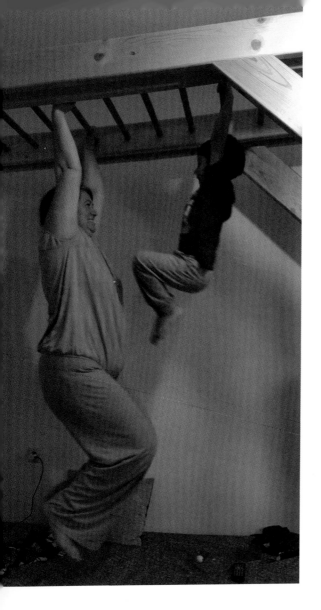

the function of the organs inside the chest. It could be that, quite simply, when you're doing something that challenges your grip strength it simultaneously challenges all of the bigger parts attached. Greater use of the hands with the rest of the upper body not only increases total movement (and total energy expenditure), it creates specific strengths and resting tensions in shoulder and chest anatomy that increase the space the organs (heart and lungs) operate within.

If that's all too technical or heavy, just think of it this way: Our bodies come with old DNA-driven technologies developed over millions of years, and the environments we're driving them in are brand spanking new. The movements *required by today's environment* might be a one-handed phone grasp and finger swipe, but the movements *required by our bodies* are based on older environments. If we want bodies to perform as best they can outside of the greenhouse and its technologies, we need to make a child's daily environment offer some of the movements it used to.

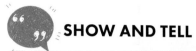

SHOW AND TELL

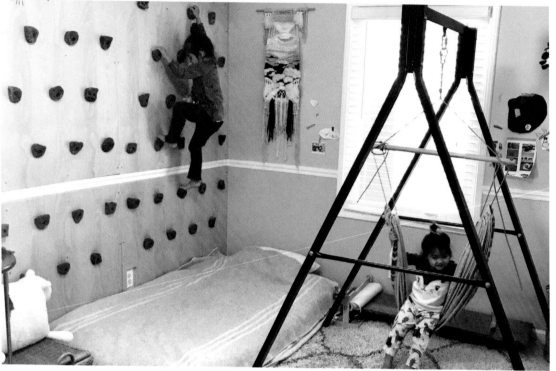

We have set up our home to increase our movement to and from the ground, as well as up above our heads. This framework of how our house can function has helped us coexist as a family of four (plus two dogs) in our 1100-square-foot space, in spite of working from home, school shutdowns, and wildfire smoke this year.

Our traditional Japanese shikifuton on the floor has become a kids' tumbling mat during the day. We promised a swing when all the playgrounds closed, adding to the clutter of their movement-rich room. The aesthetics are not for everyone, but we would probably have gone crazy (or crazier!) without these choices this year.

—Debbie Lai

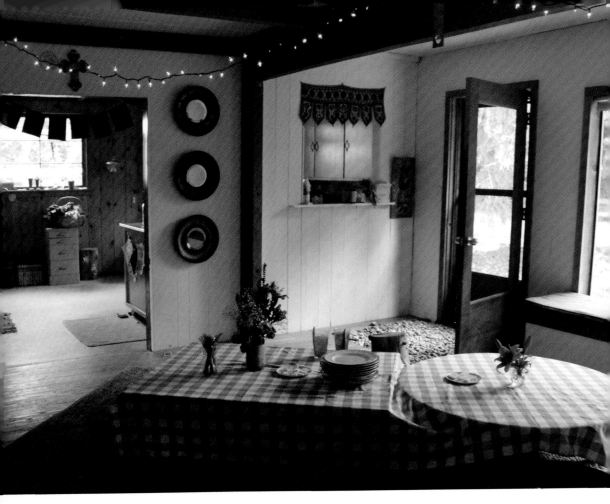

When we first considered a more dynamic home with less furniture, we thought about how others coming into our space, especially our elders, would handle it. We entertain a lot, and we figured out how to build temporary tables in our living room space (pair with twinkly lights and floor cushions of various shapes and sizes and you've got a dining room). A picnic table and benches and a couple of standard camping chairs meet the needs of those with less mobility, and a bunch of blankets can seat a couple dozen more. Flexible seating (more on that in the next chapter) allows everyone to meet their movement needs. We've even heard stories from other folks who keep a higher table and chairs in the garage for meals with family members of various degrees of mobility. The takeaway here is that most of us have been filling our houses with one shape and forcing all bodies into it. A dynamic home offers a body a variety of positions and therefore supports more movement as kids flow between them.

Take a clear look at the "movement diet" provided by your home. Is it deficient in the nutrient "upper-body movement"? Consider adding a structure that indicates and facilitates monkey-arming around. Just as growers accidently removed the movement from a greenhouse (and had to add it back in), we've cleared the trees and inadvertently kept children away from certain movements. But we can hire people to come to the house and stroke the sprouts! I mean, we can put in an arm-using space in the home that kids can engage with naturally. We can give this movement back to kid bodies so they can thrive when they're outside of a shelter.

"Tree movements" can be broken down into a variety of smaller upper-body movements that can fit into most homes. Environmental modifications do not need to be expensive or time consuming; they simply have to facilitate some sort of easy change. There is a full range of move-your-arms items, from inexpensive pre-fab pieces (doorway pull-up bars, a simple trapeze-style hanging bar and

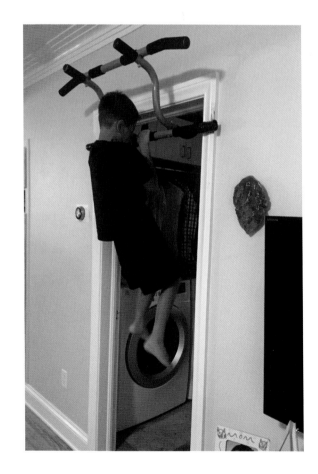

rings) to items you can build or have built.

Some terms to search for home-design inspiration and instructions:

- DIY freestanding climbing wall for kids
- Kids' doorway playground
- DIY monkey bars for kids
- Aerial silk setup
- Backyard geo dome climber
- Brachiation ladder
- Trapeze hanging bar
- Doorway pull-up bar

One of the reasons kids are often not encouraged or permitted to hang and swing is that these movements can cause injury to people and break objects when kids hang on things that aren't designed to hold that much weight. Kids have a natural affinity for hanging, so it could be there's a history of kids breaking stuff in the house, which is how we got to NO PLAYING IN THE HOUSE. As we're spending more and more time inside, recognize that we've brought more than we realize inside with us, including those natural impulses for body-stimulating movement!

Some people say that these movements are dangerous for kids even if the structures can bear the hanger's body weight. But we need to consider the problems that arise when kids grow up without the strength, mobility, skill, and judgment that are developed by monkeying around.

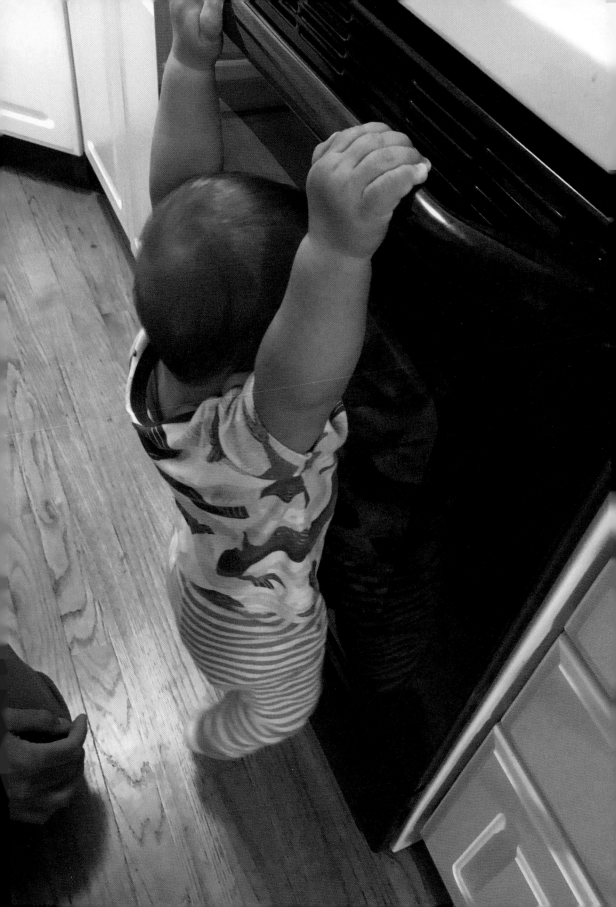

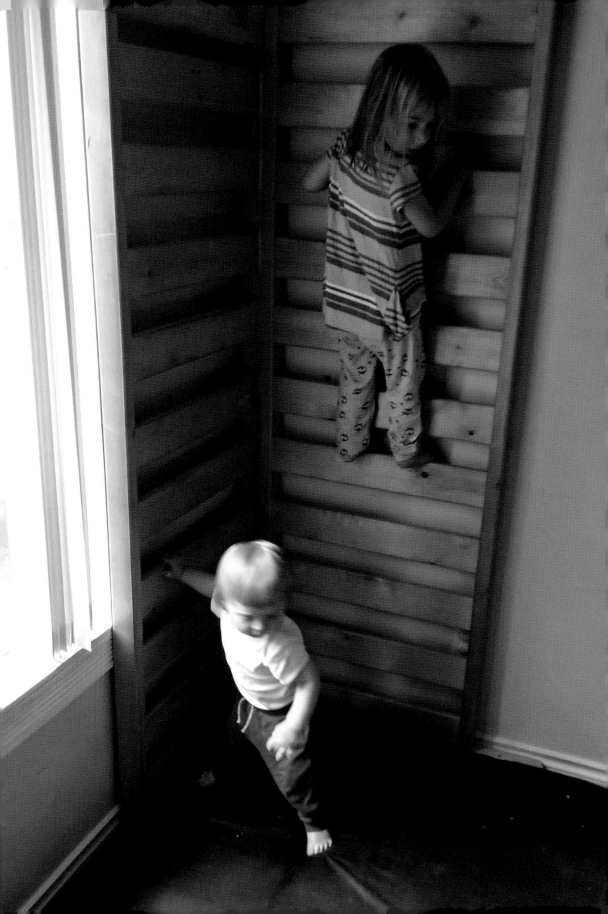

It's important to note that setting up anything for you or your family to hang on requires certain knowledge. In many cases pre-fab items come with instructions, but when you're making things yourself, reach out to local builders or carpenters for assistance to ensure you've made or hung your items correctly.

If you're not able to bring items into the home, remember that children truly just need space and permission to move in order to move their body more in their home. You can clear off a floor so kids can stretch, dance, or tumble, or you can temporarily remove precious items on display that require children to dampen their dynamic tendencies (or keep you constantly afraid of kids moving). You can clear a wall space so they can do handstands against the wall, and enjoy the pattern of dirty footprints that will gather there. There are a lot of ways to cultivate kids' reflexes to move more.

USE THE OUTSIDE PARTS OF YOUR HOME MORE OFTEN

Home isn't only what sits inside the walls of an apartment or a house; home includes the spaces that connect to the indoor parts: the patios, balconies, and porches.

Spending more time outside doesn't have to mean trips to the park or other nature-rich excursions. It can mean eating bowls of soup on the front or back steps. I'm talking *really simple* here—nothing elaborate. Getting outside is about inertia. Once you're there, the tendency is to stay there and keep on being outside. You can bring drawing and other making activities outside, create a reading hammock, and get kids out into natural light. If you have more space, you can make a fire pit, which always draws people out, or a picnic table, or a playset, or a climbing dome, or a slackline. But you don't have to.

My favorite way to build an outside-filled day is to begin first thing.

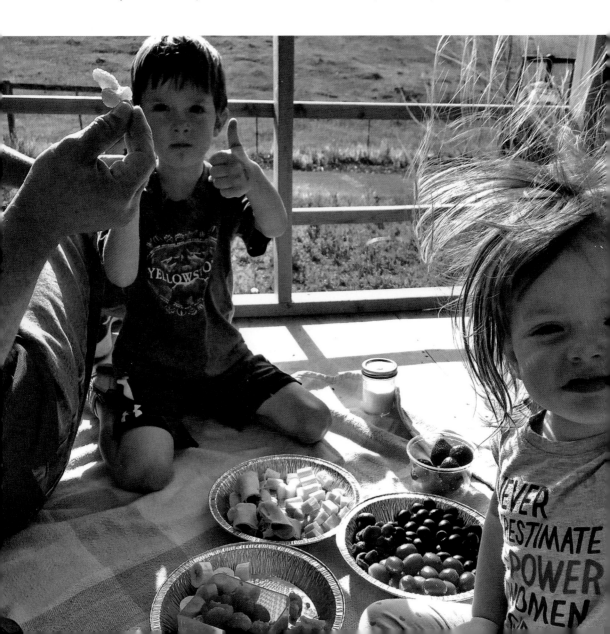

Where's breakfast? It's outside. I like to use the laws of hunger (and physics) to my benefit. Lured by food—and what human isn't?—my kids come outside, and once they're out there they tend to stay there. I was making breakfast anyway, so the only extra work was setting the blanket out. If you're wondering how to get kids outside more, make sure all the stuff they want isn't inside.

Kids, especially littles, want to be where their bigger people are. If all the stuff parents and other caretakers need is inside, then it's a losing battle. This is my way of saying if you want to get the family outside more, make sure all the stuff *you* want isn't inside, either. What family doesn't have laundry? If you're outside hanging it, they'll be outside too. After too many times of having kids come inside only because we needed to go inside to make dinner, I decided to bring my kitchen outside, a move we all benefitted from.

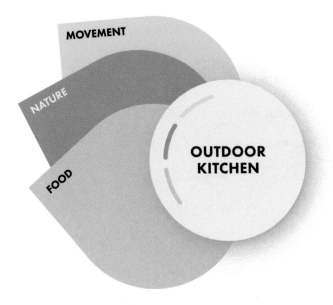

TASK: OUTDOOR KITCHEN
NEEDS MET: MOVEMENT, NATURE, FOOD

At first, I simply sat on the deck or grass chopping veggies—not only getting in some good floor movements myself, but also increased nature time. STACK! Seeing how this could increase outside time by an hour, we decided to figure out a way to stay outside longer by cooking there too. This can mean using a barbecue, getting a specialized outdoor fireplace or building a simple, safe, and inexpensive cooking ring if allowed in your area.

In addition to the structural outside elements physically connected to your dwelling, home also includes the streets, neighborhoods, and land around your home. I grew up being told to go outside. We were barely allowed inside until the sun went down. But I grew up in a rural area with lots of space and freedom to move around. This is not always the case, and more and more, there is a perception neighborhoods are not safe. Whether neighborhoods are safe or not (and many are undeniably unsafe), children who live in neighborhoods that parents *perceive* as unsafe go outside less.

That lack of safety can mean different things for urban, suburban, and rural folks. And it needs addressing by all of us. I suggest you check out one of my favorite groups working in this space, America Walks, to see how you can work toward making your neighborhood a safer place for movement. On a smaller scale, think of ways you *can* use your neighborhood safely: family walks? Sunrise or moon-watching walks? Outdoor games like hopscotch or Frisbee? Dinner on the front porch? Next time you're planning on being out, invite some neighbors to join, or offer to bring their kids along. One thing that makes neighborhoods safer is having a lot of people outside using the space in a variety of ways. You can start making that happen. Maybe reading this book is the work you're doing to get something started in your own community!

A note on neighbors: Neighbors are one more feature of a home when it comes to kids and movement. When it comes to time spent "at home" (that is, in the care of those at home, before and after school time), kids with access to safe outside spaces and a group of other kids move the most. For this

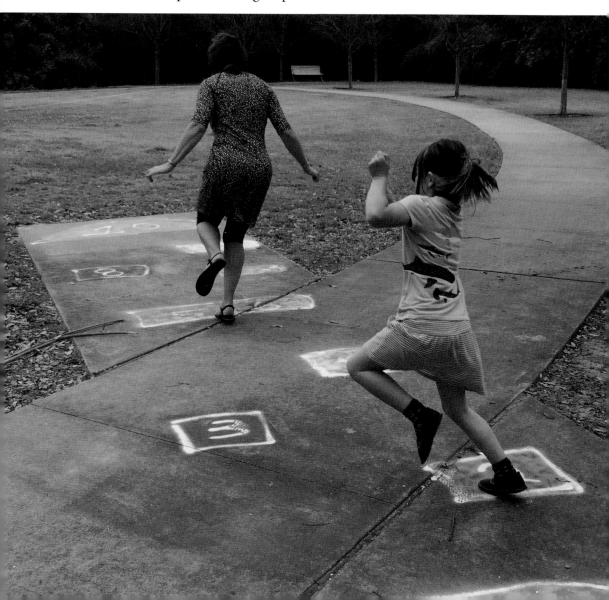

reason, building relationships with local kids and limiting the time children spend alone can increase physical activity.

BRING MORE OUTSIDE IN

It's easy to see how furniture can hold kids' body parts in place, but so do walls! There are many outdoor elements of nature (see page 45) you can bring into your home, making indoor time more nutritious.

Creating a kid-work desk, table, or reading area near a window is a simple way to set the stage for multiple interactions with nature. Windows allow for distance-looking, natural light to stream in (open for full benefit, as glass can still block certain essential rays), and varied temperatures—each of these moves parts of the body in unique ways.

INDOOR EYES

Nearsightedness (myopia) has been increasing and is now a worldwide problem. Vision can be corrected with lenses, but the myopic eye shape goes on to create serious issues in adulthood, like macular degeneration and glaucoma. Multiple studies show that the more time children spend outside, the less likely they are to develop myopia, and the more time they spend indoors and looking up close, the more likely they are to become myopic. Eyeballs need certain movements to develop well!

When our eyes focus on something up close, their ring-shaped ciliary muscles have to shorten, creating a smaller circle. These muscles are moved to their longest position (a circle with a larger circumference) by looking at things at a greater distance (think focusing on something about a mile away). Kids today are spending the bulk of their day inside, with their eyes focused on a book or device twenty inches (or fifty centimeters) from their face, or at most, across a room to a wall that is, say, twenty feet (or six meters) away.

The eye muscles are always in use, but today's indoor environments create many movements over just a small portion of the eye muscle's range of motion. This is similar to the limited range of motion modern bodies often go through at the hip: sitting in a chair and standing up and then pedaling a bicycle. Compared to the many ways a hip can and needs to move, the action of hip joints riding a bike is close to that of hips getting up and down from a chair (or toilet). Likewise, the ciliary muscle contraction involved

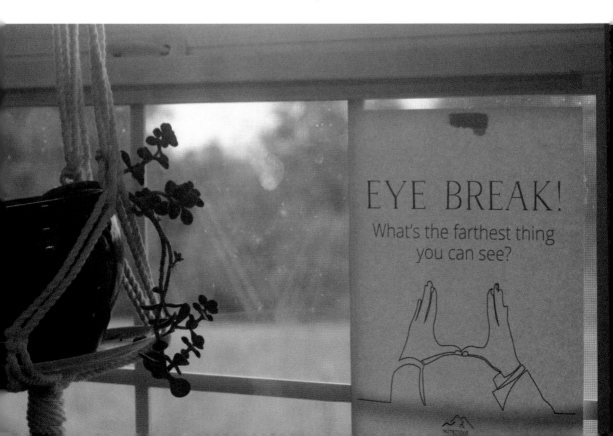

with looking at a screen varies little from that used while reading, setting the table, playing cards, or brushing teeth. And P.S. When we go to sleep, the ciliary muscles don't relax and lengthen; they contract and stay short all night long. It's like our eyes sleep positioned "in a chair"—which is why they *must* get their more diverse movement when they're awake.

Growing eyes, like other body parts, need to move as they're setting their adult shape. In order to do that, they need a lot of access to different distances and levels of light that move other eye muscles, too—ones that move the pupils into bigger or smaller sizes. Looking around outside is nature's "eye playground," and in addition to taking eyes outside more, it's important to get more of that natural movement even when inside.

It's not only for the sake of their eye health that kids need to look outside. Compared to a wall, a window offers the opportunity to observe more of and to learn more about the natural world, no matter where that window is.

SLEEPING "UNDER THE STARS"...INSIDE

My family loves the cozy feeling of going camping and sleeping on the ground. But for many, a night on the hard ground or with only a thin layer of protection is not cozy—it's a challenge and the opposite of restful. Why? Most of us are not used to sleeping on something that requires our body to move that much.

Many of our home surfaces, especially the ones we sit and lie on, have not only been elevated, *they've been cushioned*—another way of reducing the

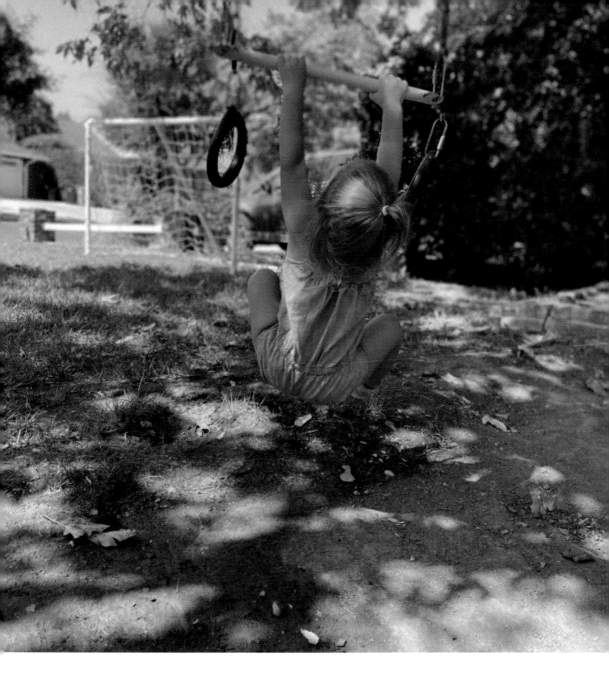

You can adjust your dynamic setup based on the weather. When it's cold or stormy, you might bring in items that allow for more movement so inside time can remain active. When it's warm, move items outside to stack arm movement with nature.

movements that happen when our body is being pushed upon (what I call pressure-deforming movements). Our bodies just aren't used to the movements necessary to deal with firm surfaces anymore.

When it came to bedding, my family knew we wanted something that moved our bodies more, something that got close to that sleeping-outside feeling. Over many years we've played with lower beds, floor beds (that wound up moldy here in the Pacific Northwest), back up to a futon, and finally back to the ground—only this time on sheepskins that have to be picked up and draped over a rail each day to supply mold-busting airflow. We've discovered that picking up bedding each day reveals a wide-open space just begging to be moved in. More movement to and from the ground, more pressure-deforming movements from sleeping on the ground, more movement setting up and breaking down the bed, and more space…all in one. Who knew we could STACK IT IN OUR SLEEP?

We busted another movement-reducing marshmallow, too: sleeping pillows. While it's almost unheard of to give pillows to young babies, our cultural norm is to issue children pillows at a young age. If you stand against a wall and place a pillow between the wall and your head, you'll see that pillows move our head *forward to the rest of the body*—a position many adults were already trying to fix before the recent infiltration of smartphones and screens began beckoning heads forward—a position young children have not yet developed.

In our house we definitely use cushions and pillows to prop us up for evening reading and movie-time, but we've forgone the all-night forward

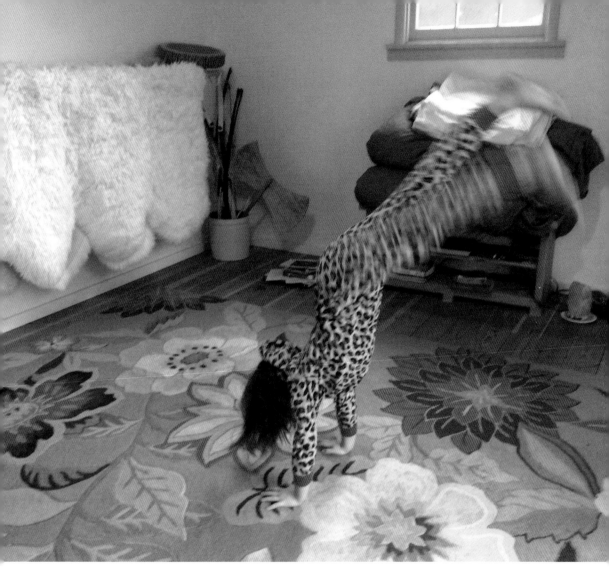

head by not starting our kids out on pillows for sleeping. It took a year to wean myself off a pillow once I realized that it was playing a role in the headaches coming from a stiff neck, and I figure it's likely easier to avoid starting on one than it is weaning off of them. (Just because the sheet set comes with a pillowcase doesn't mean you have to use it as a pillowcase. Save it for a sewing project or a sack race.)

These approaches might be uncomfortable, but only at first—and not likely for children who haven't experienced anything different. Even adults who

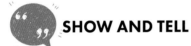

SHOW AND TELL

My husband and I live in Los Angeles, California, where our three children, aged five and younger, have spent their entire lives in an 1100-square-foot apartment. When it came to choosing a place that would allow us to move most, finding a place with high walkability was a priority. Within two miles of our apartment we have two parks, our neighborhood school, a grocery store, a weekly farmers' market, and our downtown area, where we could walk to for dinner and a movie.

I found myself craving more outdoor time for when we were at home, and noticed a long-dismissed slope of dirt, rocks, and juniper. It didn't take long before I found myself imagining what could be done to make it a functional space. I rallied the troops and proposed my ideas to our fellow tenants. After we had them on board, we brought it to our landlord, asking if we could transform this small muddy hill into a play space. Our landlord agreed to our idea, and we went to work.

With our kids alongside us, we pulled out bushes, leveled the hill with shovels, planted grass seed, and put up fencing. It became such a labor of love and source of pride for both us and our kids. That little outdoor space became more than we could have anticipated. What we hoped would be a place for more outdoor movement and rest became a gathering place. It became a place to fold laundry and chat while the kids dodged our folded piles playing tag, a place for barbecues, a place to say hello to our neighbors as they walked down the street, a place for watching someone's kids while they ran a quick errand on their own, a place our kids could create and imagine, a place to decompress at the end of the day. A neighbor who had been just an acquaintance prior to the yard became the friend and person who watched my kids in the wee hours of the morning while I was in labor with my third baby.

In short, our yard created not only movement in nature, but community. It is truly apartment living at its finest.

—Amanda Littlejohn

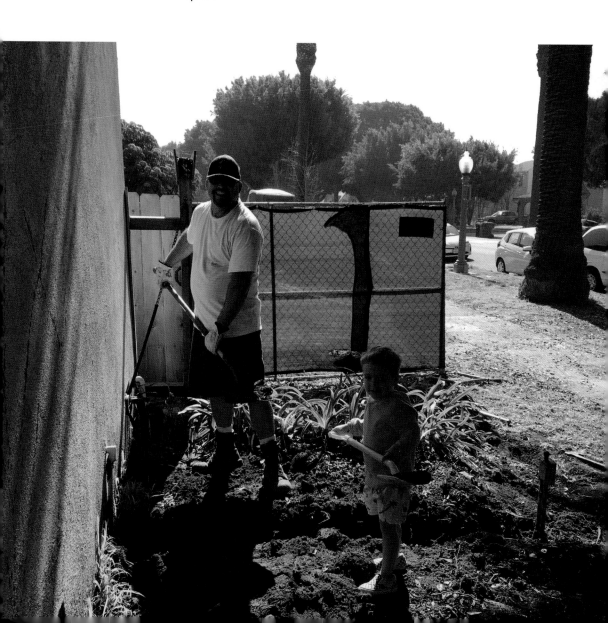

make the change soon come to find it very comfortable and start to dislike sleeping on highly cushioned surfaces. In the same way you can't feel the heel of a shoe until you've spent some time in shoes without them, we're not tuning in to the feeling of "cushioned"—because there's nothing to compare it to!

When it comes to indoor spaces we frequent, our home is likely the most malleable. Making big changes to daycare or classroom setups, for example, often involves more people and negotiation. It's a lot more work. While we are each limited by the size and shape of our individual dwellings, other variables—like which and how many things we place in our house, how they're set up, and our very home culture—are up to us. More good news: creative tinkering seems to be a human characteristic. When it comes to fashioning a dwelling that serves us better, we can put our natural strengths to good use and get to work on (and in!) a dynamic-home setup.

Our family's transition to a more dynamic home has happened over ten years. For me, it all began with my pregnant body craving the pressure of sitting on the floor. I didn't get rid of the couch, I just didn't sit on it, and it made my body feel better. By the time my first baby came, I had gotten so used to stretching out there, I brought the baby down with me and we eventually ditched the couch. (In fact, my water broke while sitting on the couch, so that might have had something to do with it. FOR SALE, CHEAP: ONE *SLIGHTLY* WATER-STAINED COUCH!)

Start with what feels easiest. A dynamic homework space? A campout in the living room with just blankets for a mattress? A living room obstacle course on a rainy day? The biggest issue is that we're not used to moving in our homes; movement is for other places. But there's no reason that has to be the case. Everyone gets to move more in a home that has both literal and figurative space for movement. Because you know those greenhouses? They're not so great for adults either.

I like comfort as much as the next person, and while our dynamic home might not be conventional, it meets our needs better than the old setup did. Our furniture and features (or lack thereof) not only give our limbs more movement taking us to and from the floor, and move all the parts of us that sit, squat, and roll on the floor, but they also create a pressure that makes it so much easier to go outside and be comfortable there. The less our house feels like one giant marshmallow, the easier it is for all of us to choose to *go outside and get comfortable.*

STUDY SESSION: SIZE DOESN'T MATTER

Home environments are changing. People are moving to more urban areas, which can often mean smaller living spaces. In other areas, average house sizes are increasing. In both cases, personal yards are decreasing or disappearing altogether. Homes now come with multiple screened devices, and often with separate areas for children and adults to use different media at the same time. Children are moving less, and researchers and designers are seeking to understand how the home environment is a contributing factor. How can the physical design of the home promote children's physical activity—or sedentary behavior—when they're at home?

One team of researchers considered the home environment's physical elements—house size, yard size, fixed and portable electronic media players accessible to children, labor-saving devices, physical activity equipment (for games and exercise)—and talked to parents. They found five "themes" affecting children's at-home movement: space of the home, how that space is allocated, equipment/furniture in a home, perceived safety of the home space, and changes in the home environment.

They found that many parents have set up a home to support more movement in the form of gear or by having fewer media devices (or by having more regulations around their use). Those with smaller living spaces have found nearby parks for more movement, and when outdoor safety is an issue, some allow "outdoor play" inside. Switching to a house full of big rooms or suddenly getting a big yard isn't a reality for most, and here's some good news: it doesn't have to be. The researchers concluded that "how families prioritise the use of

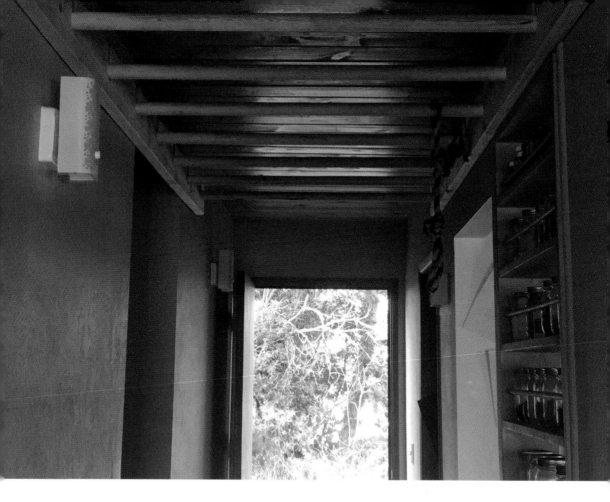

their home space and overcome the challenges posed by the physical environment may be of equal or greater importance." We just need to make movement a high priority in our home spaces, whatever that space may be.

Maitland, C., G. Stratton, S. Foster, R. Braham, and M. Rosenberg. "The Dynamic Family Home: a Qualitative Exploration of Physical Environmental Influences on Children's Sedentary Behaviour and Physical Activity within the Home Space." *The International Journal of Behavioral Nutrition and Physical Activity*, December 24, 2014.

Marmot, A., and M. Ucci. "Sitting Less, Moving More: the Indoor Built Environment as a Tool for Change." *Building Research & Information*, August 9, 2015.

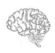 **MOVEMENT BIAS CHECK-IN: HOME**

Furniture, especially the way it is used in a Western culture, is not found in all cultures the world over and is not a very old practice. Still, having it and being upon it feels entirely normal and is even perceived to be "proper" and "what bodies need." We've probably never even thought much about it! Here are some questions to tune you in to how you feel and think about the shape of your home.

- What features of your home do you love most and why? Which parts of you are served by each feature? Are they physical or emotional?
- What features do living rooms need to have in order to be a living room? How about kitchens? Bedrooms? Workspaces? Bathrooms?
- What does each feature offer you? Would it be possible to have these needs met using a different environmental shape?
- How do you feel the features in your living room (bedroom, kitchen, etc.) contribute to you negatively? How would you adjust them if you could?
- How does sitting on the floor make you feel, physically and emotionally? If there's any discomfort, what would you need to be more comfortable, physically and emotionally?
- What rules do you have in the home regarding movement? Are they written down? Spoken? Where do these rules come from? Are there ways to modify these rules so they better meet more needs or the needs of more in your home?

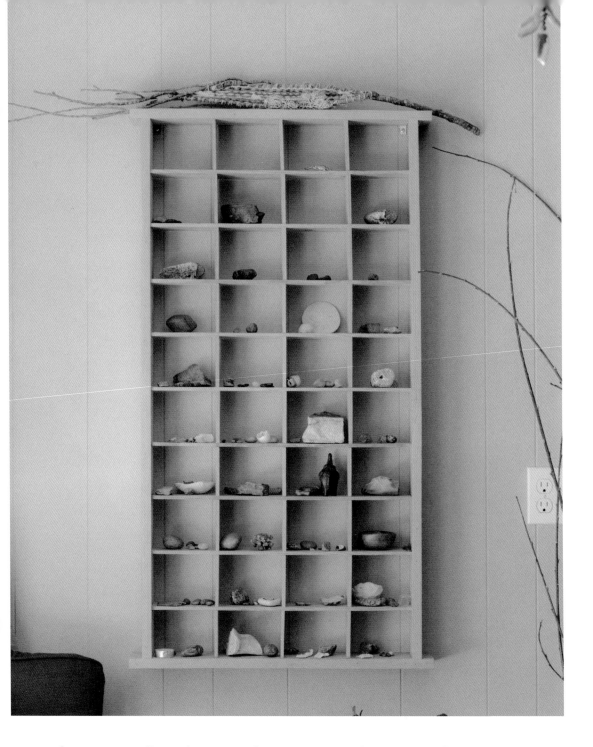

"Nature walls" make great indoor vitamin N. When your window-sills are full (see page 44), repurpose or build a shelf where you can display treasures you find on your outside adventures. This shelf is no museum; touching and handling are definitely encouraged!

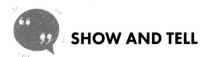
SHOW AND TELL

Authoritarian parenting has never appealed to me; since I like to understand the reasons for doing something, I try to give my kids the same consideration. When I became obsessed with Katy's work, I shared with my boys what I was learning, as I learned it, about the importance of movement. At eight and thirteen, they weren't big fans of sports or spending time in nature, but I hoped that arming them with knowledge and expressing my growing enthusiasm would help to plant some seeds in their minds. I used to joke that our family was "indoorsy," so that's where my husband and I started when transitioning to a movement-rich life.

We got rid of our seating piece by piece, lowered our dining room table, and set out fun movement accessories like a yoga ball and a balance board. A pull-up bar installed in the doorway to the computer room became a reminder to hang throughout the day. With each step we reassured the kids that we were merely experimenting and stressed how much space we were opening up for playing games, doing puzzles, and wrestling with their dad. I explained Katy's analogy comparing furniture to junk food: if you want to eat better, get rid of the unhealthy food; if you want to move more, get rid of the things that keep you sedentary. They were uncertain at first, but after every change they decided they liked things better this way. From there we worked on making family walks and beach or park outings a priority. We discovered that we enjoy hiking in winter, when bugs and oppressive humidity are not a concern. We even made a rule that we always walk the half mile to the library, somewhere we visit at least once a week. We still love what we call

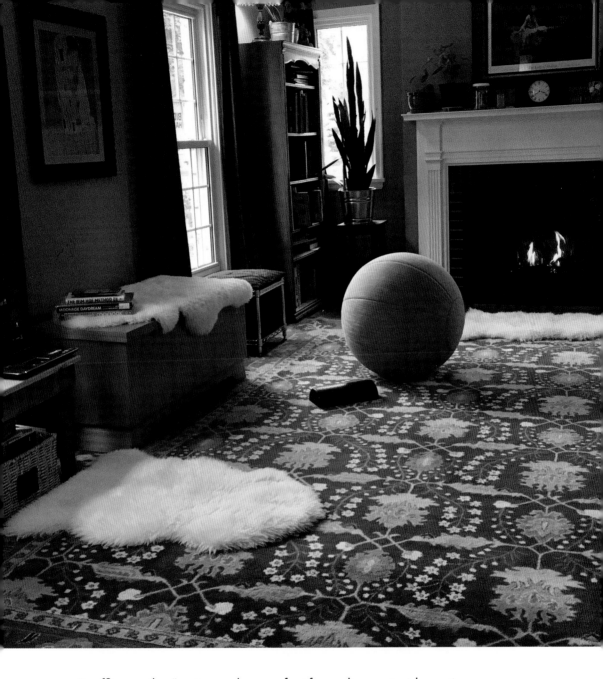

"muffin weather"—stormy days perfect for curling up inside, eating warm muffins and reading books. But through ongoing discussion and a commitment as a family, we are learning to view movement not as a chore but as an opportunity.

—Kay Ehlers

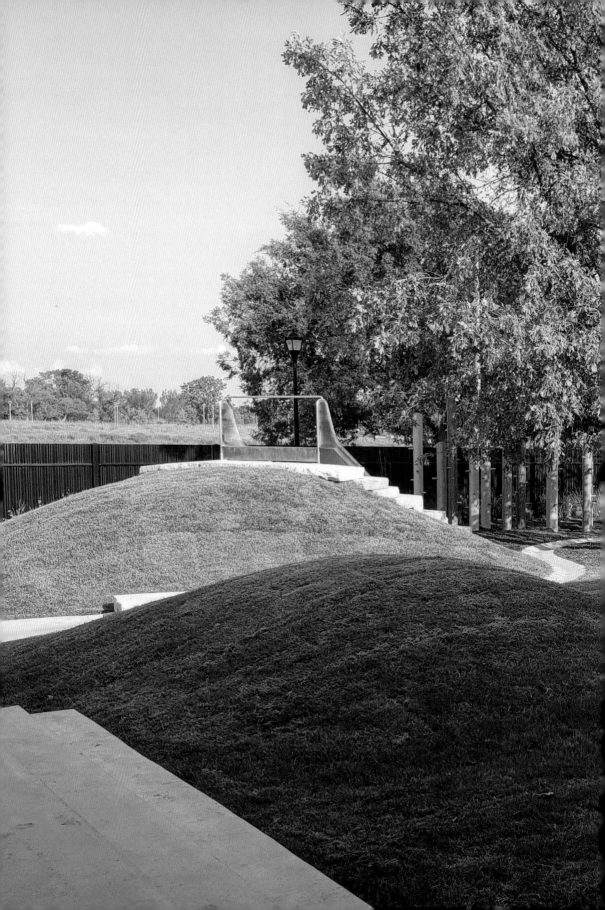

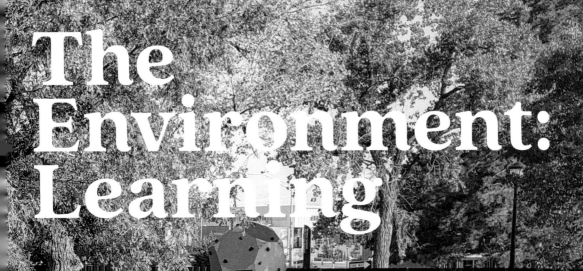

The Environment: Learning

Learning is gaining knowledge—both information and skills—through experience, study, or systematic instruction.

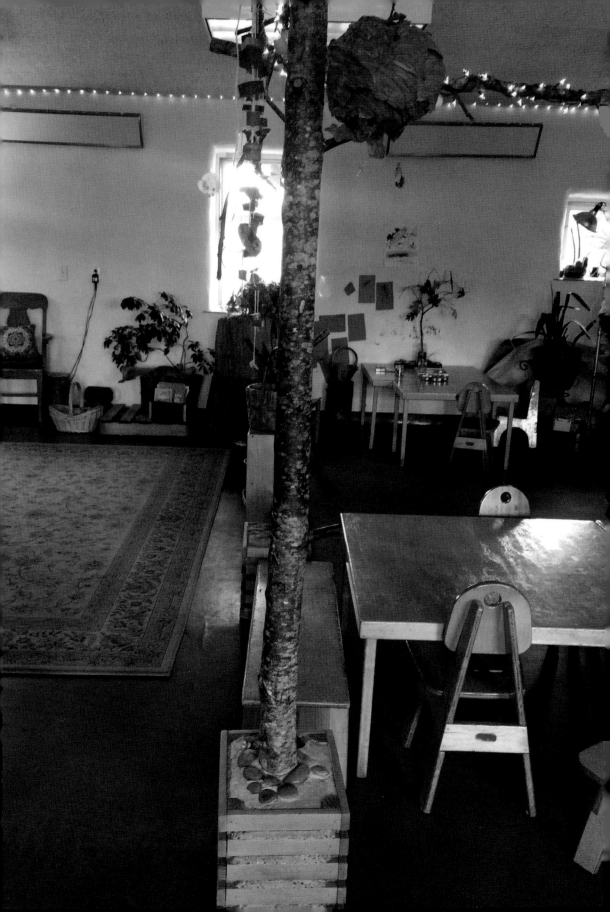

The Learning Container

Kids are dynamic learning machines. They're born into a natural world that is constantly on the move, and they're intensely drawn to it. They come with corresponding hardware—body parts that move them from curiosity to curiosity, parts that allow them to manipulate items for sensory input (how they look! feel! smell! sound! taste!), parts that deliver all of this multisensory knowledge to anatomy built for storage, and parts that allow information to be retrieved again for later use. As they gathered the knowledge and skills necessary to live in the natural world, they simultaneously gathered the movement. Kids have always learned to move by moving to learn.

But today, how and what kids learn looks much different. Just as we view nature as a much smaller environment (green spaces!) than it actually is (everything!), we've boxed learning into the much, much smaller container of "education." We've gone from "learning is everywhere" to a more formal, systematic, industrial approach to learning—*and we've put it inside a greenhouse.*

It's ironic that while "learning" is generally now indoor and sedentary, the educational environment might be the one that is getting kids outside and moving more than any other. Although the total amount of outside movement that school offers is extremely low (and is decreasing in many schools in favor of academic learning), many schools at least schedule movement time in the form of recess and physical education. In fact, simply having to get up to go to school and move between periods can increase the daily steps kids take each day.

Changing our entire cultural paradigm around education and the educational environment would be hard—likely impossible for any single individual—but there are small elements we can each work on that create change

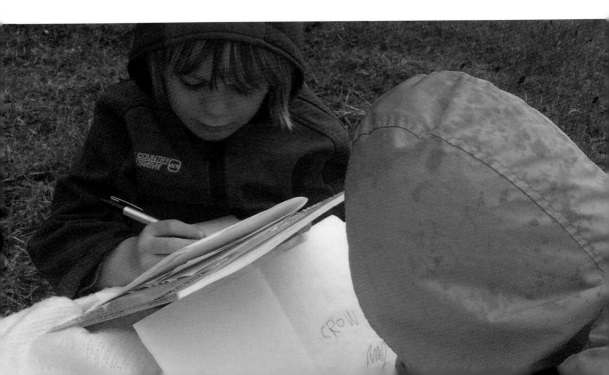

when done *en masse*. There's nothing about the learning process that says school time has to be so sedentary. In fact, much research shows the opposite. Many kids do better in school when they move more.

FLEXIBLE SEATING

The single thing kids practice the most at school isn't reading or math. It's sitting in a chair. Although this vast amount of sitting poses a problem for the body, one good thing is that small changes to the sitting environment can pay off again and again.

The concept of getting kids out of conventional chairs and desks is no longer radical; researchers have been looking at how much kids are sitting and what can be done about it. Nobody thinks kids sitting this much is a good idea, it's just that changing infrastructure—and getting so many people to start something new—takes extra time, extra money, and the ability to overcome a lot of inertia. None of these come to us easily, so it's no wonder kids are still sitting.

"Flexible seating" is an emerging concept in education and classroom design. It means that instead of the conventional classroom set-up where all the seats (and body positions) are identical, kids are allowed to position themselves in a variety of ways while they work. It's "flexible" in that kids can move their bodies more by having a range of shapes to choose from.

Dynamic seating was initially thought of as a solution for children with attention difficulties. Some kids tolerate being still all day more than others.

Kids who can't turn off their movement reflexes as easily were deemed more disruptive; pediatric therapists looked for ways these kids could be in place but not have to be still.

The provision of more physical activity in sedentary spaces is now being expanded to the wider classroom because people realized that even children who can better cope with less movement benefit from dynamic seating!

Some of the seats educators are offering students include:

- Exercise/physio balls
- Fixed or "wobble" stools
- Standing/sit-to-stand desks
- Exercise bike desks
- Carpet squares
- Bean bag chairs
- Cushions
- Benches
- Crate-seats
- Exercise/yoga mats

And remember floor sitting and squatting, which many school-aged children still find comfortable—but are at risk of losing. These positions with a low table for a desk work well, no sitting furniture required.

The transition to dynamic seating can be more complex than simply swapping chairs (see sidebar on facing page). For parents, this means asking teachers what support they would like in order to make this change and how

MOVEMENT BIAS CHECK-IN: LEARNING

Adding dynamic seats in a classroom is like a single twist to a Rubik's Cube: one move mixes everything up! The procedures of education spaces often depend on everyone being still. If the unexamined Rule Number One of a classroom is *"nobody move,"* educators might not realize that they need to adjust some of their teaching methods along with the chairs. Making a sudden switch to a more dynamic learning environment can create chaos and the false appearance that all-day sitting is better. For a sounder transition, here are some questions to ponder.

- What movement rules, explicit and implicit, do you have in your classroom? Could these rules be revisited and revised with the students to help them tune in to the movement environment they might not be aware of?

- What needs (and whose) are met by staying in a chair? Could these needs be met in a different way?

- Kids are often inexperienced in being allowed to choose how and when to use their bodies, and need assistance to navigate this new option. What guidelines would help them? What guidelines would help you?

- If kids are moving, their stuff needs to move with them. What other items in the classroom might need to change?

- How could students be involved in transitioning a space from being sedentary to dynamic? How can this become an opportunity in core skills (e.g., what lessons could involve measuring/evaluating personal movement before and after, creativity, communication, collaboration, problem solving, making/building)? What would this teach them about movement, the malleability of environment, and meeting more of their own and another's needs?

you might contribute. For education professionals, this can mean starting a conversation with the school administration to figure out what would be needed to make this change, how you might contribute, and how to get parents and students involved.

Seating is one environmental change that takes little work once the transition is made, but there are other ways to get a classroom of kids moving. Outdoor classrooms—which don't require specialized structures but simply move students outside, perhaps utilizing campus greenspaces that are only being used at recess—can be used for a lesson or a period. Lesson plans can be created around movement. One of my favorite lessons as a student in-

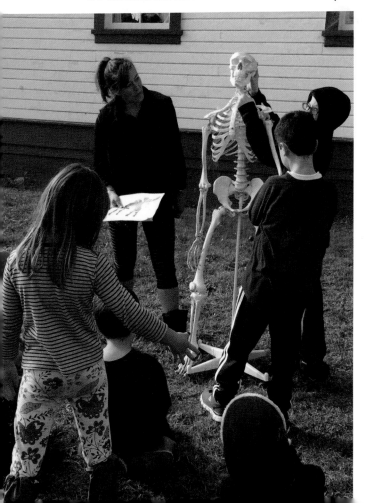

volved calculating our own horsepower (search "human horsepower lab activity" on YouTube) by timing each other running up a set of stairs. Another teacher has her class "act out" the prepositional phrases—"behind the chair," "under the desk," "with my friends," "in the middle"—as they learn them.

There are many ways to stack core curriculum with

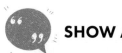

SHOW AND TELL

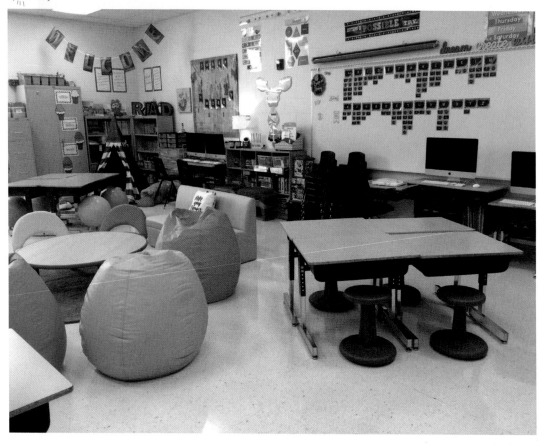

As an occupational therapist in a school setting, I've observed that adding extra movement within the school day seems beneficial for many children in the areas of attention, participation, and work completion. Some classrooms are converting to a flexible seating arrangement, which may include choices between standing desks, floor tables, wobble stools, floor pillows, and exercise balls. Additional movement options include desk and floor rocker chairs (e.g. Virco), balance boards to stand on, and balance chair cushions.

—Elizabeth Gudenkauf

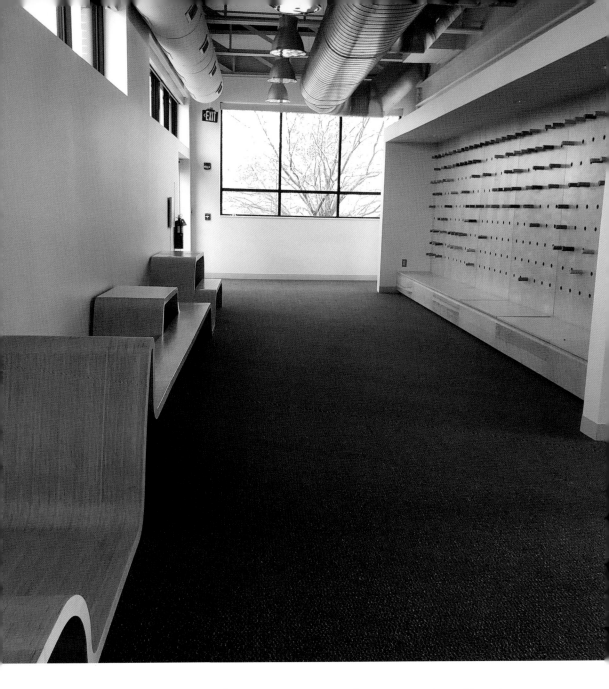

Designing spaces for more movement is becoming a thing. This photo is from Wonder, a microschool in Kansas, designed with the intention of facilitating more movement outside of a movement class. The hallway wall and its pegs are not only where school bags can be hung; they double as a playful movement feature, where kids can hang from the pegs as they move themselves across the wall.

walking. In programs like The Walking Classroom, students listen to specialized podcasts for 25-minute walking lessons and then engage with their teacher about what they've learned. Measuring, journal writing, and many science topics are easily transported outside. The possibilities are endless; they just require thinking about how to add movement to concepts that are being taught.

PHYSICAL EDUCATION AND BEYOND

Without much movement in daily life, we've put learning about movement into a specific class at school. Physical education (P.E.) is a course you can find in many schools that's designed to improve how children move. During P.E., kids practice specific movement skills and learn the rules of various games. They perform bouts of athletic exercise or play a sport. But the movement they get during structured, directed classes tends to be different from the way they move during periods of self-guided free play. Recess and free play include explorative, diverse, and playful movements that can bring about experiences with nature and others that are often absent in traditional P.E.

Both P.E. and free play have their place. It's helpful to have time set aside to hone a movement pattern and learn the intricacies of a sport, team dynamics, and performance. But research also shows that children need blocks of time where they use movement as a way of exploring the seemingly non-movement parts of the world. In short, developing bodies need nature play.

P.E. class grows up to become exercise. Exercise is great, but perhaps an unintended consequence of a kid having P.E. as their primary (if not only) movement experience is that it can lead them to believe that the only purposes of movement are performance, athletics, or exercise. Those who don't like performance, athletics, or even games may come to believe that movement is not for them.

Many schools have movement teachers—teachers who probably love movement themselves and have a passion for getting kids to move. These folks probably already advocate for more play and recess time for kids. Just like teachers interested in shifting to flexible seating, they would undoubtedly appreciate your support for more free play opportunities, especially for younger children—ask them how you can help! Even alerting them to the fact that you care can be encouraging.

For those who design curriculum, remember that exercise, dance, and sports are a much smaller subset of all the ways kids can move and will need to move as adults. Green up movement time by including adventure walks, scavenger hunts, and "nature games" (see examples in the next chapter). These not only deepen the movements found in a P.E. session, they can be part of the non-P.E. curriculum too. All teachers can add movement; kids need to move more often.

Finally, look for opportunities to tune kids in to the movement that can happen in between classes. Simple line-balance challenges of chalk, paint, or tape can be placed in hallways with a sign: "Can you walk this painted/tape line and not fall off?" Let them know how far they're walking: "This hallway

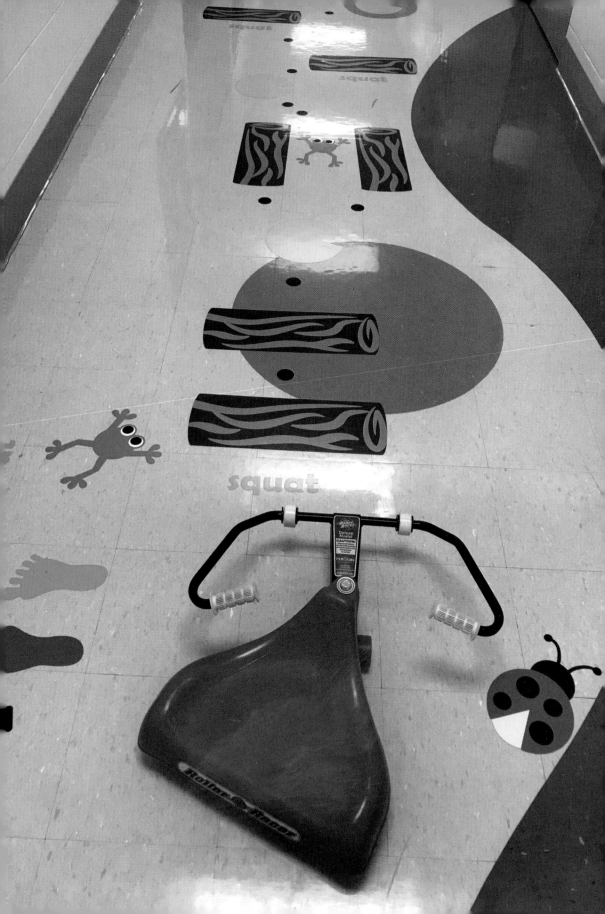

is 48 steps long" or "The library is ⅛ of a mile from the cafeteria," "The walk to school from the parking lot is 1 kilometer." Teach them about the carrying they're doing and how to do it better: "How heavy is your backpack? Weigh it here!" "Try carrying your backpack in these four different ways!"

Right now, nobody is teaching kids about all the places movement belongs outside of exercise. That's probably because those kids are growing up in the care of the only group of people ever to have moved less than today's kids: today's grown-ups. Our culture demonstrates to its children that movement happens in class with a teacher, that it fits into a short period of minutes-per-day, and that it is for games. There's no mention of labor (moving for the things you need) or active transport (using your body to go places). Yet this awareness is sorely needed, for these non-game, non-play parts of adult life are where we find enough movement once we grow up and leave school.

Kids need to learn that their environment holds the potential to be dynamic and that they're expected to move through it. They need help being moved at first, but the goal of movement education—my approach to movement education—is to teach them how to see for themselves the opportunities to move more, as well as to ensure they have the skills necessary to take those opportunities. The education container can be made over with little change in infrastructure. Have them do the measuring. Let them make the signs.

SCHOOL MOVES FOR LIFE SKILLS

Danielle Hughes is the lead teacher at a private school in Oregon—a school that serves children with unique learning differences, focusing on students impacted by autism spectrum disorders. Below she shares how she has layered movement into an existing curriculum. She is also the co-founder of the Paeonia Foundation, which is dedicated to providing services to the autism community, and where movement, functional skill building, and therapeutic environments are encouraged.

I am a lead teacher of a classroom of individuals severely impacted by autism. I work with teenage and adult learners who have (for the most part) had a very sedentary life. There is an emphasis in our culture on "fitness." In special education, fitness is presented as *the* way to break a sedentary life and also address problem behavior. While there is some research showing that people with autism who regularly increase their heart rate experience a decrease in the frequency of severe problem behavior, it must be individualized. We are also looking to teach life skills that will be maintained in our learners' futures. We know that based on their preferences, traditional fitness in a gym will not continue by choice in their lives past school. However, if we embed meaningful movement into an activity that becomes a lifelong preference, their movement will be maintained. At least that's the hope.

My classroom focuses on life skills, independent-living skills, leisure (activities/hobbies), finding our learners' preferences, and communication. Many people, autistic or not, are used to (and comfortable with) sitting. You do one activity and then you sit, you learn sitting down— who learns standing or even moving now? Well, my class does now.

We hear from parents who go on walks in the woods or take a vacation to the beach that their child is off balance, and it is frightening. The hours walking on a treadmill to improve their "fitness" have not applied to their walking in real life for family outings, and those events are what really matter.

And so we work movement into all our activities. While we do the dishes, we stand on uneven ground. We start with a sand surface but work up to a rocky mat.

After reading *Move Your DNA*, I immediately knew we needed to move EVEN MORE, and with even more purpose. We've positioned highly preferred items really high or on a lower shelf. We have a step stool to reach what we need to make our coffee. Our silverware is on the bottommost shelf in our kitchen area. When we do stickers or paint, I hang the blank canvas on a window or high on a wall, so learners are required to reach higher and extend their range of motion (while motivated to do their preferred activity).

We go for barefooted walks in the morning and experience different textures on our feet, all for a purpose: we need to check on our garden, we play Frisbee on the grass, we need to walk across the wood chips and onto the pavement to get the basketball. Getting our feet wet just means we can get even more movement. Sitting down to dry our feet, having to sit on the floor in a new position to even reach our foot, standing up with different support, putting our socks on from the floor (not a sitting typical chair), requesting help, doing more laundry if our socks are dirty...the list goes on.

For lunch, we have a small table closer to the floor so that we can sit in different positions while we eat. While some educators may say that sitting on the floor is not age-appropriate for adults, I disagree. Not only are we teaching varied movement, but we are also teaching that you can eat in different locations.

Introducing a garden club has been so rewarding. Students participated in building a raised garden bed (for learners who are physically unable to bend down safely) and one that rests right on the ground. Creating our garden stacked meaningful instruction onto movement onto art onto participation. We built, painted, filled with soil, and planted seeds. Every day we are able to increase our duration of time spent in the garden! We bend down (in a modified squat...sometimes using a chair) to weed and pick our vegetables. We then work on standing up out of the chair or from the ground without pushing on our own body or the surrounding environment. We carry varying loads of buckets, water, soil, and compost using both hands and in different ways. And when we pick our vegetables, we go inside to cook them, teaching our learners that there is an end product and that we benefit from it greatly.

We also try to choose active field trips. We go apple picking, play Frisbee at the park, walk around a zoo or in the woods, and eat lunch on the grass or the dirt. Field trips are a perfect opportunity to model for learners and their parents how you can stack movement into your child's day without them even realizing.

While I know typical educators may not have a garden or grass to walk on, they can easily reorganize their classrooms to make the most-used items slightly out of reach, or at least harder to get to. They can vary where and how they sit during the day, including on the floor. There is no law chaining students to a desk...so MOVE!

My final note to teachers: encourage varied movement, don't be afraid to have your classroom look different, and remember that students' time in your room is shaping their bodies for the future.

ADD NATURE TO EDUCATION

No matter what they're doing, no matter which environment they're within, kids are gathering and processing what they are exposed to. They are always learning about the world around them. The question is, what part of the world are they being exposed to?

For practical purposes, we've put all learning inside the greenhouse. The learning environment used to be rich with nature, movement, and community; now learning involves very little nature or movement, and simultaneously, our knowledge of the world outside the greenhouse is shrinking.

Many schools have little to no access to greenspaces. Still, natural elements—plants, natural light, ground sitting, natural learning materials, and fresh air—can be brought into a classroom, just as you can bring them into a home. Some schools, recognizing their students' need for green and growing things, have converted sections of paved-over school ground into gardens. Change can feel overwhelming, but one way of cutting through that feeling is to start by making a list of what is needed. Through that simple process it becomes clear that a small step—like adding a plant or opening a window— is an immediate possibility.

ADD NATURE EDUCATION

Movement is not the only thing missing from the way our children now learn; knowledge of the natural world is also missing.

Science class is the portal to learning about the natural world, and while

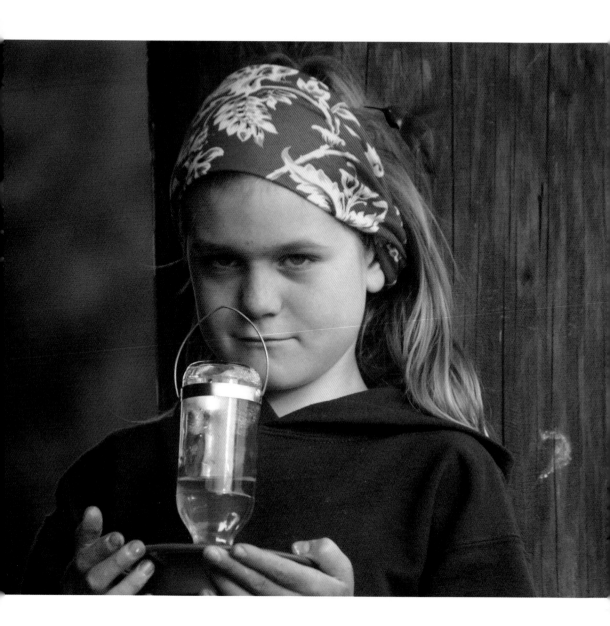

Needs: Nature, learning, nature learning, movement, community

Stack: Spend an afternoon figuring out how to become a hummingbird feeder (hint: red headbands go a long way!)

I loved it (the moon rocks coming to my school in third grade were part of why I wanted to be an astronaut, which then led to how bodies work in space, which then led to how bodies work, and now here I am writing this sciency book), scientific knowledge is not the same as knowing how to be nature.

At least at the child level, science consists of looking at elements of the natural world outside of the context these elements typically occupy and operate within. Some lessons are hands-on, like growing a bean plant in a paper cup, but many are not: learning the water cycle from a book while never going outside to test what water in the air (or not) feels and smells like, or learning the parts of a muscle cell from a video but not moving our bodies to experience our own muscle contractions. In order to teach children about

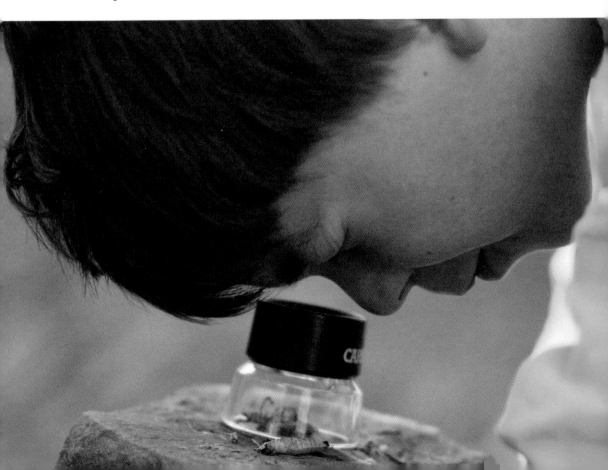

STUDY SESSION: DO TEST SCORES GROW ON TREES?

Backpacks. Calculators. Pencil sharpeners. These are some school tools, but what about trees? Learning about nature, even hands-on nature learning, does not require lush green spaces. Still, studies looking at academic performance and "greenness" have found that kids do better in schools that are surrounded by trees.

In the United States, schools are functionally segregated. Richer neighborhoods and schools have more greenery around them, and urban, low-income schools have almost none. Could this disparity account for some of the inequality in academic achievement? Researchers have found that this is indeed the case. Children perform best academically when there is tree cover within 250 meters (820 feet) of the school.

Contact with nature has also been shown to be associated with better health, lower stress levels, and less violence and crime. Psychologist Ming Kuo and her colleagues point out that adding trees to a school campus could be a low-cost investment with ongoing benefits. It's also worth considering that underprivileged schools are often the ones less likely to have recess, i.e., time to move outside with the trees.

Kuo, M., M. Browning, S. Sachdeva, K. Lee, and L. Westphal. "Might School Performance Grow on Trees? Examining the Link Between 'Greenness' and Academic Achievement in Urban, High-Poverty Schools." *Frontiers*, September 25, 2018.

Kuo, M., S. Klein, M. Browning, and J. Zaplatosch. "Greening for Academic Achievement: Prioritizing What to Plant and Where." *Landscape and Urban Planning*, November 3, 2020.

nature, we've tried to bring it to them as they sit in the greenhouse. As with P.E., studying nature in this way is a natural extension of how our society is set up.

Learning, nature, and movement were once all bound together—they were side effects of being immersed in a more natural environment. When you depend directly upon nature, there is no option but to move as you learn to use it properly.

In some ways, technological advances—from digging sticks to satellite imaging, from snares to electron microscopes—have revealed to us more elements of nature than hundreds of thousands of years of immersion in it could ever reveal. But the incredible detail of that knowledge is held by relatively few people. Simultaneously, the knowledge required to successfully be in green spaces has diminished nearly to the point of extinction. Very few humans still hold the knowledge necessary to survive in nature without the aid of a massive set of nature-consuming technologies—knowledge that every human being once had to hold in order to survive.

This is all to say our education container is missing the vital lessons of how to care for ourselves—eat from, shelter within, manage our general needs—in wilder environments. Nature learning is a stack—it's a return to learning in the way humans are used to learning—in which the natural environment provides many of the lessons found in core curriculum books and children are free to move and play as they experience them.

Many parents are now turning to "nature schools" to offer their children

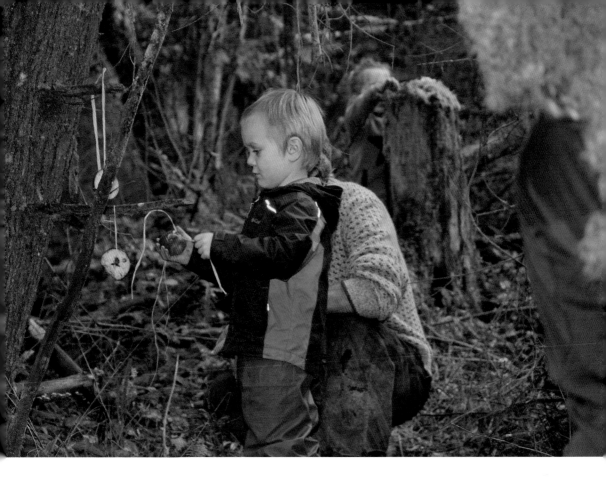

this broader way of learning. There are a variety of such schools—nature pre-schools and forest kindergartens, outdoor grade schools, wilderness immersion programs for teens, and even parent/infant hangouts in green spaces.

Not all nature schools are the same. Some teach conventional "core" academics outside, some use a nature-centric curriculum, and others are a hybrid. There are also options that fit in outside of traditional school time. You can find nature education via afterschool or weekend programs, and nature summer camps. You can also DIY a nature curriculum—there are many books (*Forest School Adventure* and *Urban Forest School* by Naomi Walmsley and David Westall are great books to start with) and online instructions, and some nature instructors share free tips and lessons via social media. If you also use your library for resources, nature school doesn't have to cost a thing, and it can be a way to stack movement and nature learning into the non-school parts of your day.

Outdoor schools aren't the only way children can learn how to better connect with nature. Any teacher can expand their indoor curriculum to include more nature in the form of the stories and books they select, the materials they use, and the lessons they create. Movement is not the only thing that slots into a lesson plan—nature can too! It can be as simple as swapping out marbles for acorns. Bringing out-of-the-greenhouse elements into the greenhouse is like stroking plants—it's a solution that meets us where we are.

Kids have become trapped. As mentioned before, many schools set aside a period of time for getting kids to move, and parents have learned to depend on an education system to teach their kids to move. Movement, however, is not viewed as a "core skill" from an educational standpoint, which makes recesses and P.E. classes easy to cull in exchange for more academic skills kids will *really* need in the future. Unless movement is stacked back into education—more dynamic sitting, academic lessons outside and on the move, a curriculum that includes the natural phenomena children will continue to depend on—movement and nature will keep being viewed as dispensable *by an entire culture*. As a result, they will continue to be systematically removed from this society, and technologies that attempt to compensate for their absence will continue to be built. Kids have become trapped because their movement depends on their adults' ability to move, which is greatly diminished. We adults have to move first, and then, like a Rubik's Cube, we have to be able to move along with each other as we collectively shift the shape of how our culture learns.

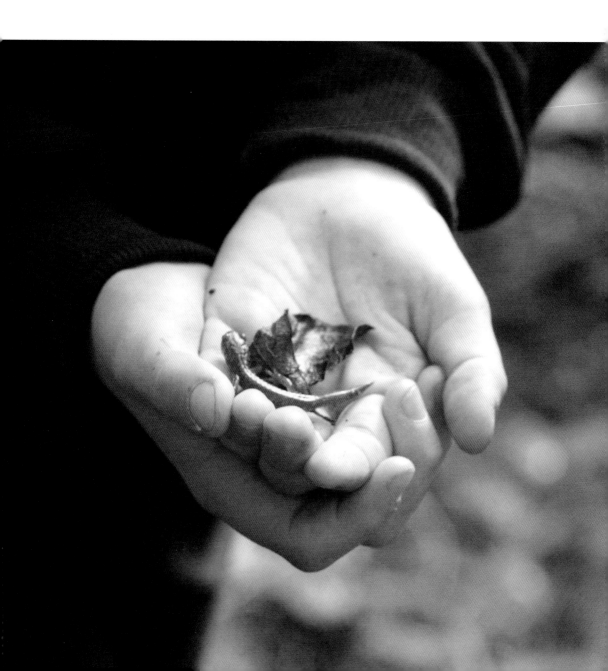

ALL-DAY MOVEMENT IN SCHOOLS

Movement coach Annette Cashell is passionate about getting schoolchildren moving more all day. She has developed a program called Movement Month in Ireland that helps teachers, volunteer fitness professionals, and parents worldwide introduce their kids to lots of school- and body-friendly ways of moving. Learn more at movementmonth.com.

School settings can feel insurmountably sedentary, but there are very simple ways we can introduce movement into schools.

The Movement Month program helps teachers, movement professionals, and parents introduce a new movement idea to the class every Monday, and explore it in depth for the rest of the week, for four weeks. Each theme focuses on a skill or habit that can be applied throughout the school year and is aside from dedicated physical education classes.

The Movement Month themes are Sitting Less, Sitting Differently, Going Shoeless, and Movement Breaks. Every day, children try new ways of moving based on that week's theme, and by the end of the week they have learned a range of moves that keep their bodies active and their minds engaged. Teachers have noticed a change in how children pay attention in class—although they wriggle at their desks with express permission, they're also focusing better on their work.

Movement doesn't have to always be a break from work or a disruption in class. Movement is in fact a vital way for students to learn, and can enhance sedentary lessons. Many can learn how to support teachers adding movement into their class!

WALKING SCHOOL BUS

Remember I told you I was going to talk about walking? School is a great place to fit in a walk. If you can't walk the whole way, drive only partway. If you've got a lot of time, great, but even a handful of minutes can be a great chill after a hectic morning of "would you *please* just eat your breakfast?" and "where have all the socks gone? SERIOUSLY!"

Eat breakfast along the way if it frees up some time. Take other people's kids if you can, to reduce the whining and make it more exciting. This all works after school too, although I'd recommend including snacks then. Kids are often exhausted after school, but not from using their bodies. It's the opposite. A snack and a walk makes a great transition—a place to replenish their dietary and mechanical nutrients at the same time.

And "school walks" aren't only good for getting there and back. We've done lots of homework on foot—practicing times tables, memorizing the lines of a school play to allow kids to tie their brains and bodies together—in the evenings and on weekends. You can even make walking the lesson by doing a family or community walkability assessment (find a link to a Walk Audit Toolkit in this chapter's references) to see how your neighborhood/school route measures up.

Dynamic, nature-rich learning and homework that moves us all, and can help shape a community? Now that's a stack!

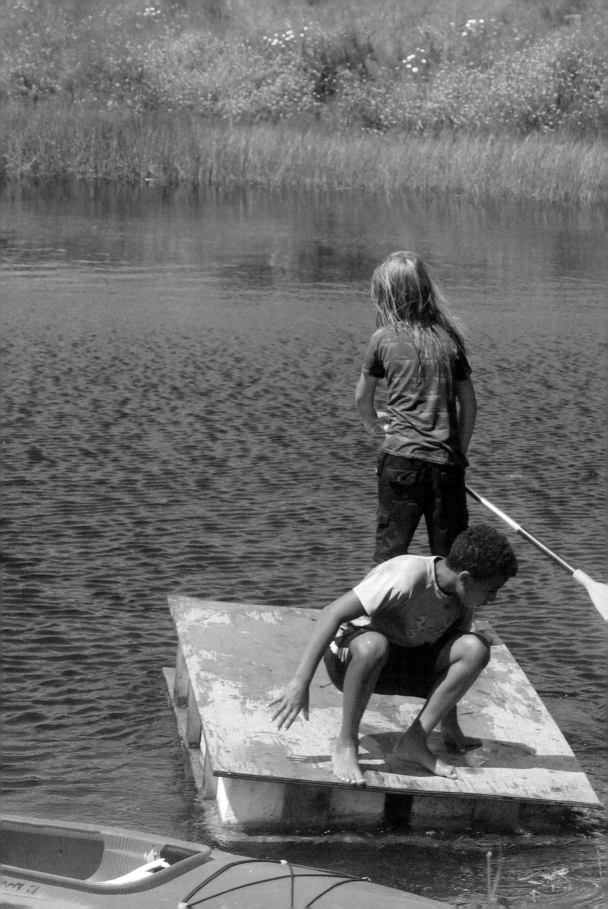

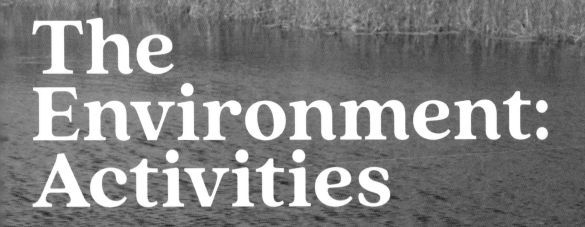

The Environment: Activities

Activities, as in "extracurricular" or "after-school" activities, are pursuits that offer a period of movement, play, or learning (and sometimes all three).

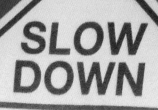

SLOW
DOWN

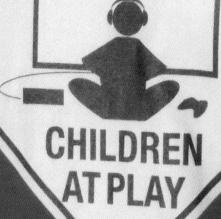

CHILDREN
AT PLAY

The Activities Container

A ctivity time is everywhere: before and after school, during weekends, on holidays. Activities are pursuits that offer a period of movement, play, learning, or some combination of the three. They can be formal (lessons, perhaps even paid for, led by a facilitator) or informal (gatherings for play or learning that kids just fall into on their own, perhaps adult-led but also kid-led). There are formal activities that offer movement, like sports or dance lessons, and those that are more sedentary, like music or language. Informal activities, too, may or may not include movement. A gang of kids riding their bikes through the neighborhood, pickup games of soccer in a local park, and practicing cartwheels and tumbling on somebody's lawn are all active examples. Reading, drawing or painting, working on Lego solo or in a group, gathering around to watch another kid play a video game (or coming together virtually while all playing online) are more sedentary informal activities.

CHILDREN'S ACTIVITIES AND THEIR MOVEMENT DIET

There is such a long buffet of activities to choose from that the "activities container" can be a tremendous source of movement and a great place to round out a child's movement diet. In order to do that, we need a way to evaluate the quantity and qualities of movement an activity fosters so we know which movement nutrients kids are getting and which they aren't.

Saying "kids need to move" is like saying "kids need to eat." Both are entirely correct statements, but they aren't specific enough to be very helpful. Kids need to eat *a range of foods that provide them with the right amount of nutrients*—calories, macronutrients (fat, protein, carbohydrates), and micronutrients (vitamins and minerals). In order to thrive, kids need to consume this range of nutrients by choosing (or being given) a range of foods that contain them. Similarly, kids don't just need to move enough (e.g., for a certain length of time or calorie expenditure each day); their bodies need *specific* mechanical nutrients. In order to build a nutritious movement diet, we need a way to tell which moves make which nutrients.

In order to become a chemical reaction in your body, food must be put into your mouth. Sunlight starts a chemical reaction by shining on your skin. Movement creates internal chemical reactions by bending and squishing the

cells of the body. Each movement bends and squishes the body in a particular way. There are many technical ways to quantify and qualify movement,
and many of them require knowing a lot about how each body part can be
moved. But to keep it simple, start by observing which of your kid's body
parts are moved by an activity. What body shapes and positions are they
using? Do their activities require lot of leg motion, but not much arm movement? Do they spend a lot of time using their hands but not much else? Are
they using their core muscles for balance but keeping their arms and legs still
(think riding a surfboard or Onewheel)? Kids can help figure out which parts
of their bodies they use during their activities. Have them list their top five
activities and show you the motions they use for each. Write them down. You
can create a chart: head, eyes, neck, shoulders, chest, arms, elbows, wrists,
hands/fingers, spine, waist, torso, hips, knees, ankles, feet, toes. For each activity, have them demonstrate which motions are used at each of these parts.

If the cells that are moved are the ones creating the chemicals, then it is
these moving parts that are being most nourished. You can use your "which
parts are moving" analysis to sort activities by which body parts are moved
(and bonus: kids are now clued in to the concept of observing their own bodies and body parts as they are active).

But wait, there's more! When it comes to part-by-part movement nutrition, we also have to consider the body parts that aren't as easy to see, like
the heart, lungs, bones, and eyes. How do we tell if these parts are moving?
In short, by thinking of what moves them. For example, the cells of the heart

and lungs are moved by other body parts moving more. Moving the body fast (i.e., getting the arms and/or legs moving *vigorously*) is one way to move the heart and lungs. Another way to get the heart and lungs moving is by carrying something—a backpack or another kid or even yourself up a tree, up a hill, or across the monkey bars. When looking at a list of activities, you can add "moves heart and lungs" by looking at the speed of motion, if there's an increase in a load being carried, or if the body itself is being hauled up or lowered down. Kids can also report if it makes them huff and puff! P.S. These situations not only add heart and lung movement, they also increase the movement nutrition of the limbs doing the increased work.

Bones are another hard-to-see body part, and there are good reasons to pay attention to how they are moved during childhood. As kids mature, their bones are not only growing, they are being formed. Bone mass, bone density, and bone shape are being set throughout childhood and early adulthood. These bone attributes largely determine a person's peak bone strength (resistance to fracture) and the upper limit of their bone density. An older person's susceptibility to osteoporosis is so strongly influenced by the quality and quantity of their childhood movement, osteoporosis is regularly referred to as "a pediatric disease with geriatric consequences." Osteoporosis prevention begins in adolescence. The dietary nutrients (especially calcium) *and* mechanical nutrients a child experiences don't guarantee strong bones in adulthood (adults have to keep moving to maintain them), but a child's food *and* movement diet set the upper limit of how strong their adult bones

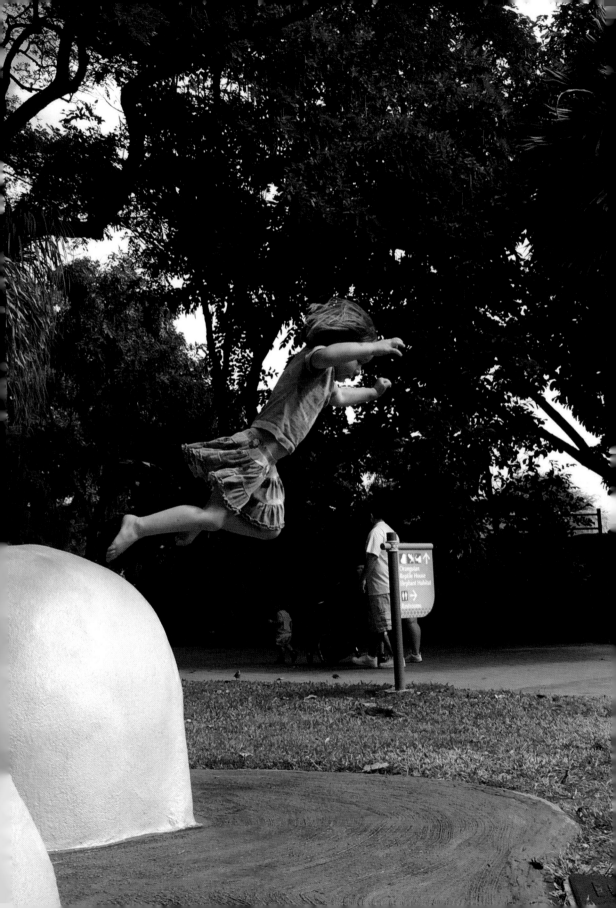

can be. We've already discussed some specific movements and how they can affect bone formation in the face and jaw (see breastfeeding "playground" on page 153), hip and leg bone formation (see baby positioning on page 221), and shoulder bone formation (see hanging on page 230). When it comes to activities, we can assess how they move bones more generally by evaluating how "weight bearing" an activity is, or how much body weight the activity places on the skeleton.

Let's consider a few activities in the light of these suggestions. A kid could swim two hours each day, which will move their arms and legs vigorously, and move their heart and lungs too. However, the body is pretty weightless in water, so the bone cells don't get squished. Swimming is nutrient dense, but it doesn't contain all the movement nutrients kids need. Bicycling is another movement that gets the legs, heart, and lungs moving a lot (but only through a small range of hip motion; see sidebar on page 324), but it's done mostly seated, which again doesn't give the bones—especially the hip bones—the body-weight loads they need to grow strong. Standing on a skateboard causes the body to bear more weight than sitting on one does, but there's not much impact involved.

Walking and running are body-weight-bearing *and* they both create bone-squishing impact with each foot strike. "Impact" means that for a brief movement the load created by your body is higher than your body weight. And speaking of impact, jumping is great at building bones for just that reason. The high impact upon landing a jump is a brief "super-squish" that lets the bones know they need to beef up. Bones need impact to maximize their strength, which is likely the main reason kids are naturally drawn to jumping up and down on things (let's hear it for innate body wisdom!). Their body needs this movement to build up the less visible tissues of bone, ligaments, etc., and jumping is the "food" that gives them the movement nutrients their tissues require. What sort of bone loads do the activities you're considering offer?

Finally, eyes, as previously discussed (see page 246), move more when they are focusing over a range of distances (looking at the same distance means eyes aren't moving as much) and when they are used in natural lighting. How do the activities you're considering move a kid's eyes? Are their eyes getting any of the movement nutrients found in natural light? Are their eyes having to use only up-close looking movements, or does this activity offer a variety of distances (and thus a variety of eye movements)?

By going through this process, you will have a framework to assess how activities are currently moving your kids and to identify which specific body areas and tissues might be undermoved. P.S. You can do the same with your own activities; it's likely you and your kids need the same movement nutrients and can get them together!

STACK YOUR ACTIVITIES

Kids have a tremendous number of body parts that need to move, and most of them need a *lot* of movement. Right now we've culturally allotted very little time per day for movement and we try to "move kids" by picking activities to fill in that small amount of time. How do we meet multiple part-movement needs in one unit of time? We stack it, and give kids the activity (a.k.a. "the task") that moves them the most and in as many ways as possible.

For example, jumping doesn't only move a kid's bones. It also moves the heart and lungs when done repeatedly in quick succession, as in a game of jump rope or when trying to master a jump off something high enough to provide a thrill. It also moves the hips, legs, knees, ankles, feet, and even the arms a bit.

But movement isn't the only thing to be reaped during a period of movement. In addition to moving all the parts, jumping makes you good at jumping—and at landing well! Jumping off stuff, for example, can add confidence and cultivate the ability to explore areas that require knowing how to better handle your body. The jumper naturally learns to judge distance and the stability of the landing surface. They might need to take turns with others and figure out the best way to clamber back up to jump again. An activity can hold more than movement nutrients; it offers practice and eventually the ability to perform a new skill.

Fundamental Movement Skills is another framework for kids' movement. It focuses on "gross motor development," which is the ability to organize the use of their large muscles to get their whole body from place to place. This framework categorizes the movement skills children need into three categories:

1. Locomotion (walking, running, skipping)
2. Body control (stability and balance while moving)
3. Object control (manipulating, carrying, throwing, catching)

A "balanced movement diet," then, would ensure that skills are developed in each of these categories.

Other folks working with kids use a physical fitness framework. Because there is a correlation between physical fitness and health, the idea is that a kid's movement diet should meet these criteria:

- Cardiovascular endurance
- Muscular strength and endurance
- Flexibility
- Body composition
- Agility (how quickly they can change the direction they're moving in)
- Balance
- Coordination
- Speed
- Power
- Reaction time

Which framework is right? They all are. Kids need all of this stuff—to move all of their body parts the best way and the best amount, to develop all of their body-brain programs (motor skills), and to develop all of the movement skills that their adult bodies might want to call on in the future—and the corresponding health and well-being that comes with getting all of the movement their body needs.

And here's the final stack(s). Kids need to move all their parts in all the ways *and* develop all their large *and* fine motor skills along the way, *and* meet their physical fitness nutrients, *and they need lots of outside time and community—specifically, to move with other people, including other kids.*

The scientific process has revealed a long, itemized list of "what kids need," which can feel totally overwhelming to parents and others who care for kids. But don't let the details generated by this pursuit of knowledge overwhelm you. **A short list of simple, inexpensive, and natural kid movements has been meeting all of these needs in a stacked way for hundreds of thousands of years.** This is the original stack: grow up moving for many hours every day, thereby becoming physically skillful and successful in nature in a small, then medium, then full-sized body. The movements involved are part of our kids' genes. They include walking, running, sprinting, jumping, ground-sitting, wrestling, carrying (and being carried), climbing, throwing, catching, swimming. The original stack involves doing these movements

 SHOW AND TELL

Our eldest has just reached a stage where she loves to play with older kids (and will leave us be when she does). We've noticed that during those interactions her movements are more varied and sometimes reach a higher level of difficulty, which no encouragement from us will produce. There is also a lot of joy. We try to maximize play opportunities with kids of varying ages by going to parks more often on weekends, during school holidays, and arranging play dates with friends with older kids.

—A. Do

over a variety of uneven surfaces and in a variety of weather, moving around things like other kids, moving quickly, with barely enough room (have you ever noticed how a bunch of kids playing on a crowded, elevated platform on a playground run around each other coming *this close* but not knocking into each other?). It's balancing on branches. It's throwing rocks. It's jumping down off something again and again and again.

These movements are stacked because as a set they provide all of the body parts with the movement (mechanical nutrients) they need to develop well. In addition, they fulfill all the needs listed in the proposed kid-movement frameworks, and they develop the physical relationship we need to be in and move successfully through green and wild spaces.

GETTING THE ACTIVITY DIET IN ORDER

Activity time isn't only for meeting kids' movement needs; activities can also meet kids' needs for community, play, nature, and learning. This is an additional way to assess and choose activities. How much community are their activities offering? Nature? Education? Nature education? What about play? Are all their activities structured, or is there balance provided by informal activities that offer freedom to explore movement and knowledge in a self-directed, *more playful* way?

By taking stock of your activities, you might find some that can be swapped out for those that are more movement-centric or provide different nutrients. But because every family has their particular culture, sometimes it won't work to swap out an activity. Not to worry. Like many containers previously discussed, the activity space can become more dynamic by changing up the way an existing activity is being done. Adding flexible seating for seated activities or transporting an "indoor activity" outside adds movement.

All activities add something arguably beneficial. The approach here is to discover which movement needs are not being met by looking objectively at how kids are spending their activity time and how they're moving during that time. You can then swap stationary activities for ones that offer more movement and outdoor time. Or if kids are doing a lot of *one* type of movement-rich activity—say a lot of swimming, biking, or a single sport—you can swap some of that time for another activity or two that gets more parts moving. And don't limit yourself to considering only formal activities and how you might adjust them; it is likely the informal activity time—when kids are sitting around the home doing the same activity again and again and again—that will be easiest to change. DID I SAY EASY? I meant simple. Simple means uncomplicated, but not free from work, work that's often repetitive and done over a longer period of time.

HARDENING OFF

When plants destined for the outdoors are grown inside, they need support to transition outdoors for best results. Plants need to develop certain anatomy (like leaf cuticles) to thrive outside, but that anatomy is only developed by *being* outside. So if seedlings are grown inside, gardeners and farmers "harden

SHOW AND TELL

I'm a piano teacher, so my work with kids mostly happens after school hours. After a day of being cooped up in a desk and a room, kids don't need more practice sitting still, but piano playing is hard and takes focus. It's hard for me to be still, too. There's not a lot of room here in my studio for vigorous movement, and I don't have time to make movement separate from the music lessons. What I've done is make movement okay in this context. I have a big ball for either of us to sit on or lie on or wiggle around on, balance boards, many active music games that involve getting up and away from the piano, maybe squatting or lying on the floor or what-

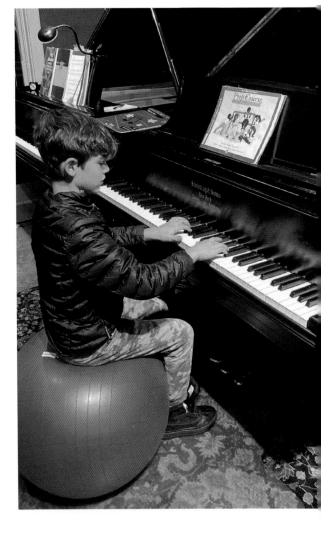

ever. If the kid is wiggling or jumping up, I do the same thing. You can stand up to play the piano, sit on the ball (it's quite a challenge), kneel on the bench, jump around between tasks. We both need it, it normalizes movement in lessons, and it makes it possible to teach kids in the afternoon and enjoy it. My friends who don't teach this way complain of discipline problems, poor focus, and lagging interest, which aren't problems around here at all.

—Megan Hughes

them off" by gradually exposing them to the elements. This means putting them outside in a protected area that gives them a low dose of outdoors to stimulate their outdoor anatomy to develop. Growers have to watch the weather and choose when to bring the seedlings back in (sometimes it's too windy or snowy to put their fresh bodies out), and they move them back into the greenhouse for a cozy night. The seedlings can stay out for increasingly long periods of time as they become better built for nature in a stepwise way.

We aren't used to thinking of kids as being built for sitting inside, but right now, for many, this is the main experience they've had. Dragging them away from the environment they've grown in and planting them outside for hours doesn't give them the opportunity to be successful. We adults have been mostly raised in a greenhouse and aren't sure ourselves when to go out, how to find or create that "sheltered nature," and how long to stay out in order to avoid overload. Adults can better convince themselves to be outside and move around "because it's good for us," but that mostly doesn't work for kids. This is why small doses of being outside and gentle movement—patio picnics, an easy family or class walk, building a snowman, or a game of sidewalk hopscotch—are simple ways of getting started. Bringing movement tools into the greenhouse, like a low box in the living room and permission to jump off it, can be great ways to harden off.

Once kids get over their inertia, and once they have the anatomy that allows them more movements, their natural desire to play physically, bend to explore, hop from rock to rock, gather shells and stones, and climb trees can

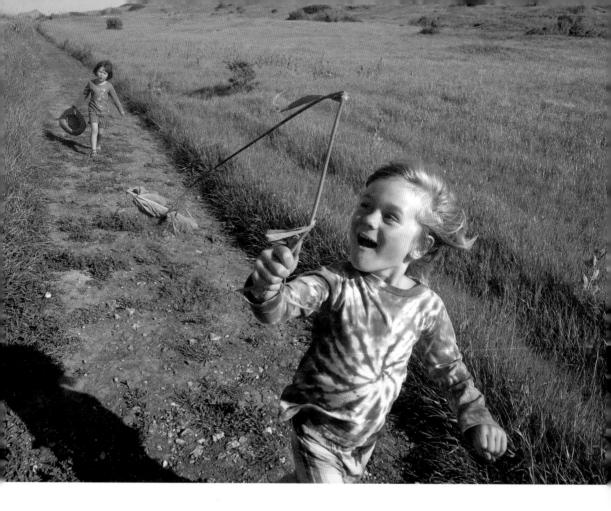

kick in. The more they are absorbed in being outside and engage in a slowly expanding range of movements, the more they'll get better at being outside and doing even more movements. They will gain momentum. Again this process is not complicated, it just takes them time and for their "growers" to harden them off thoughtfully.

It can often seem that children's activities require specialized manufactured (and often expensive) buildings, equipment, and outfits. But in reality, the movement- and nature-rich activities that meet children's needs are so old that they originally required no purchased equipment. It didn't exist!

Here are some activity ideas organized by "skill."

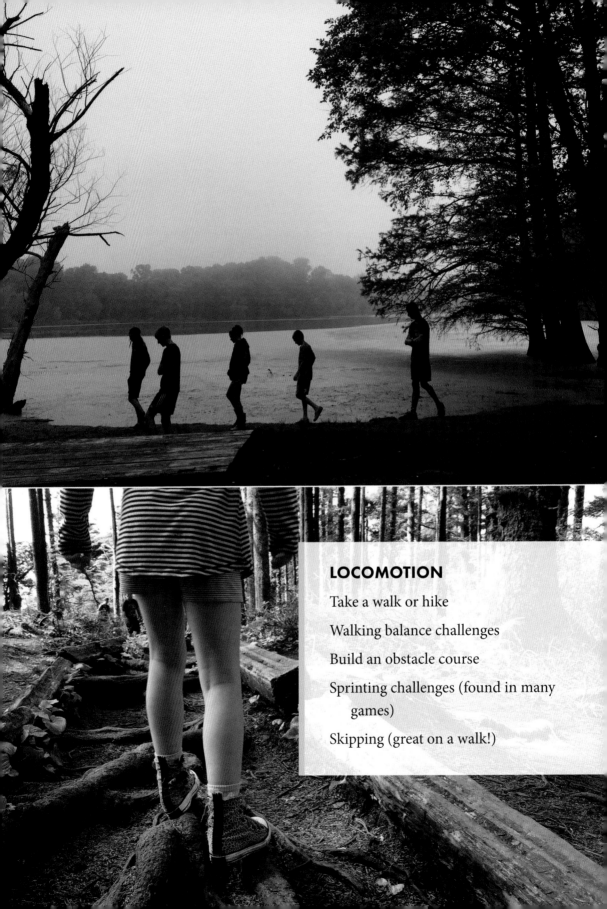

LOCOMOTION

Take a walk or hike

Walking balance challenges

Build an obstacle course

Sprinting challenges (found in many games)

Skipping (great on a walk!)

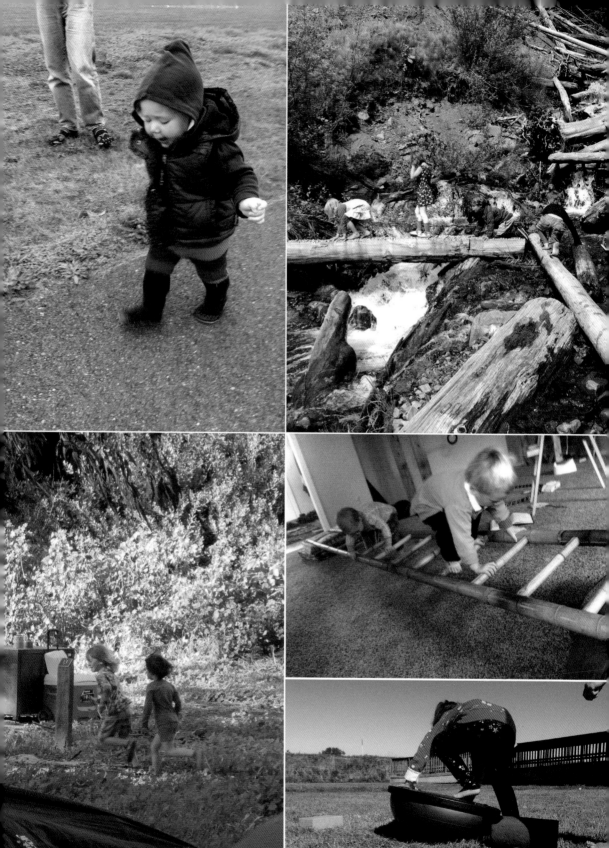

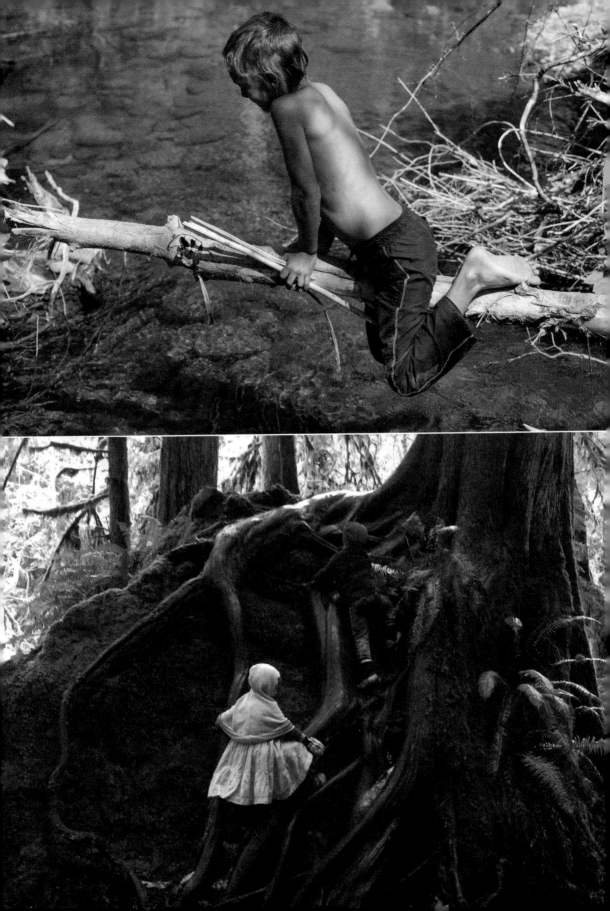

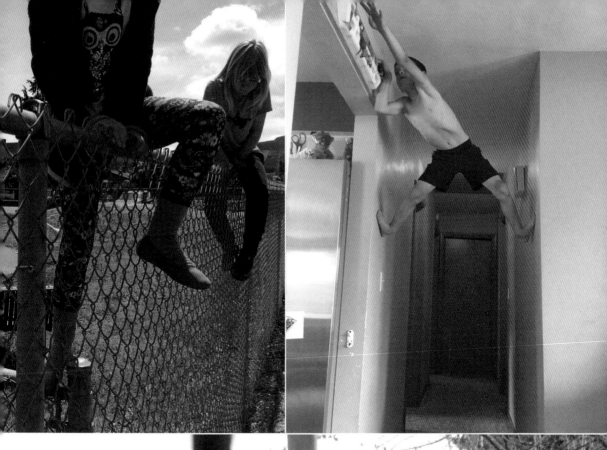

CLIMBING, CLAMBERING, HANGING

Play on hanging station

Visit park monkey bars

Climbing walls or boulders

Find a neighborhood "climbing tree"

Encourage off-road clambering—over

  fences, railings, etc.

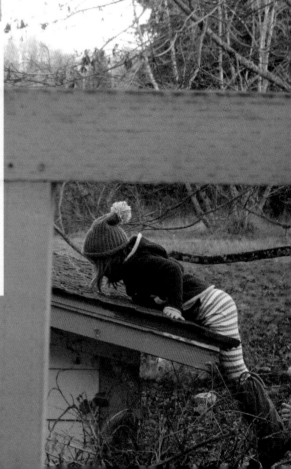

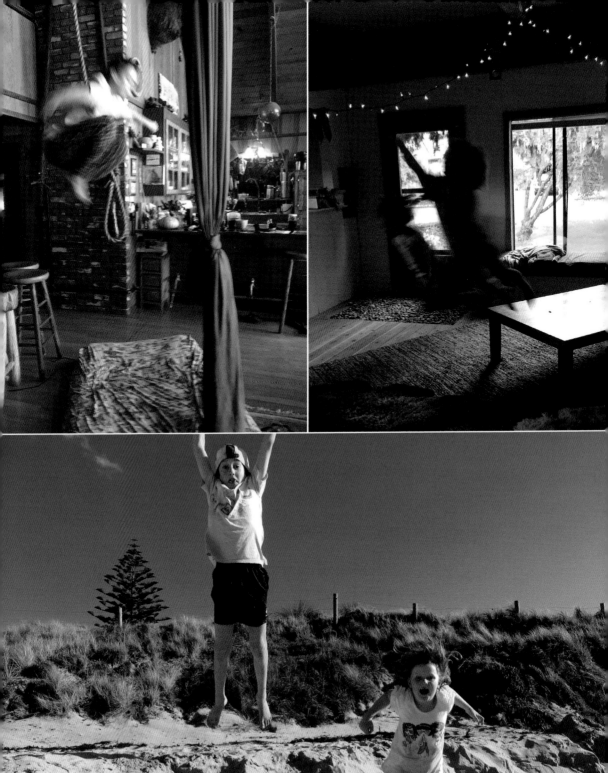
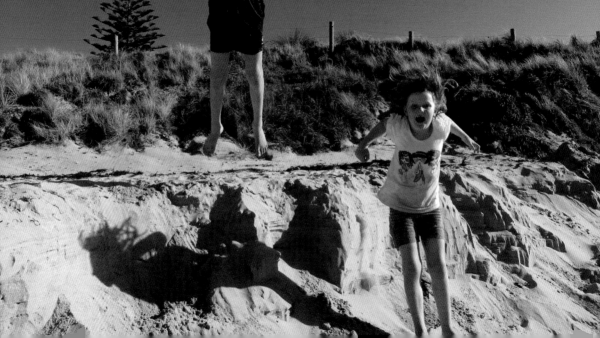

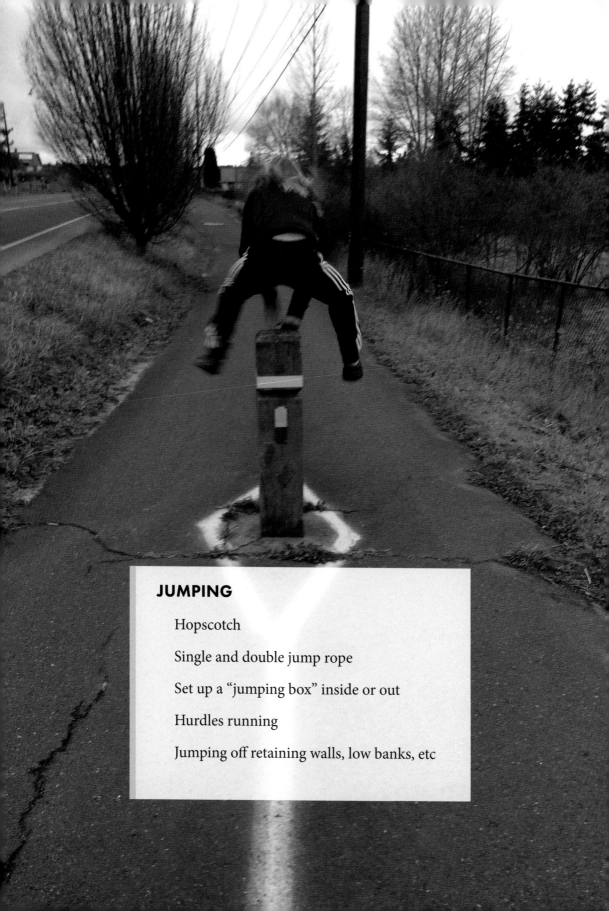

JUMPING

Hopscotch

Single and double jump rope

Set up a "jumping box" inside or out

Hurdles running

Jumping off retaining walls, low banks, etc

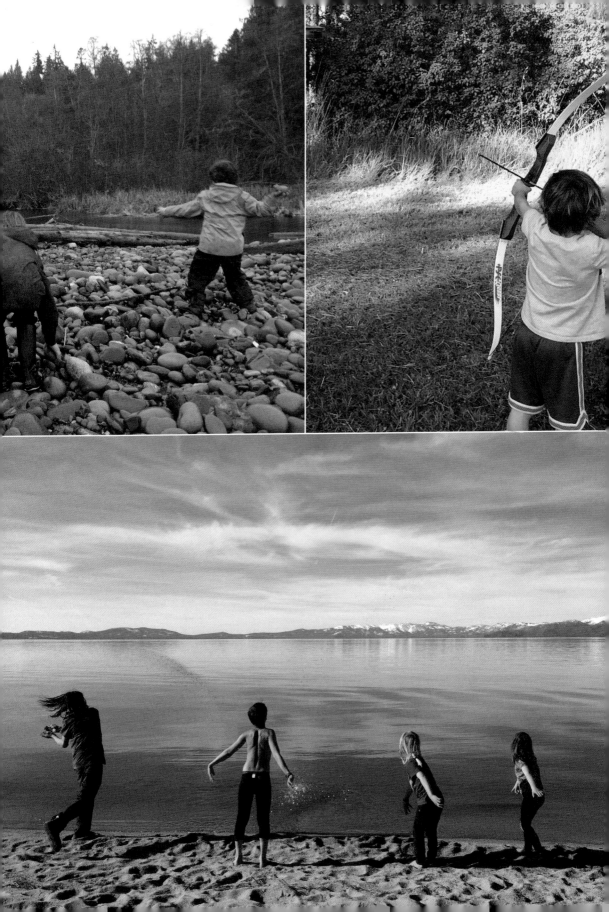

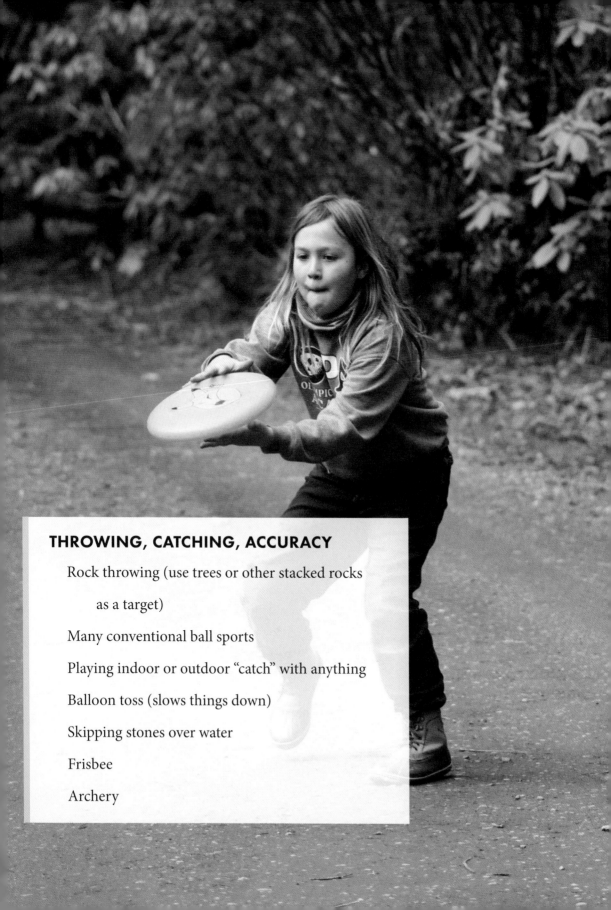

THROWING, CATCHING, ACCURACY

Rock throwing (use trees or other stacked rocks
as a target)

Many conventional ball sports

Playing indoor or outdoor "catch" with anything

Balloon toss (slows things down)

Skipping stones over water

Frisbee

Archery

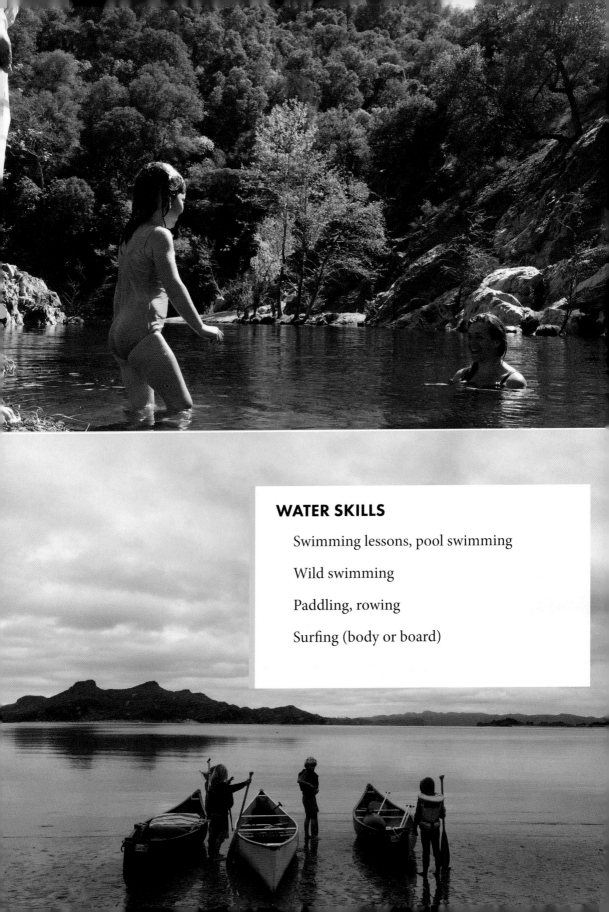

WATER SKILLS

Swimming lessons, pool swimming

Wild swimming

Paddling, rowing

Surfing (body or board)

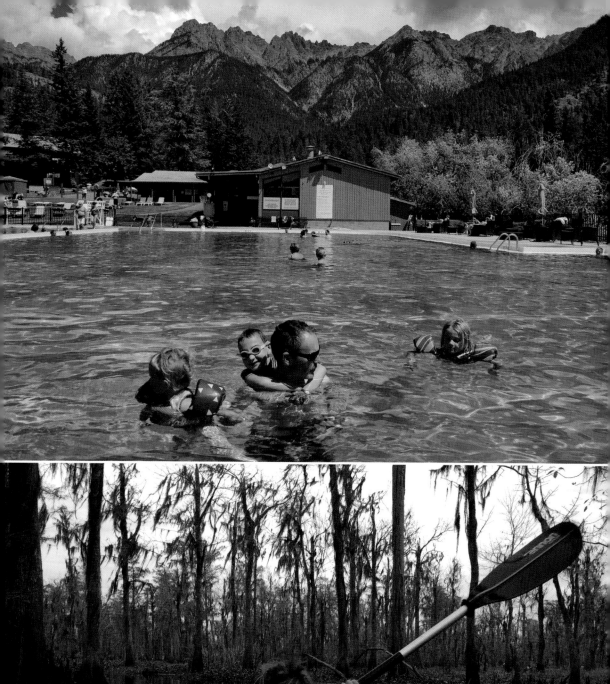
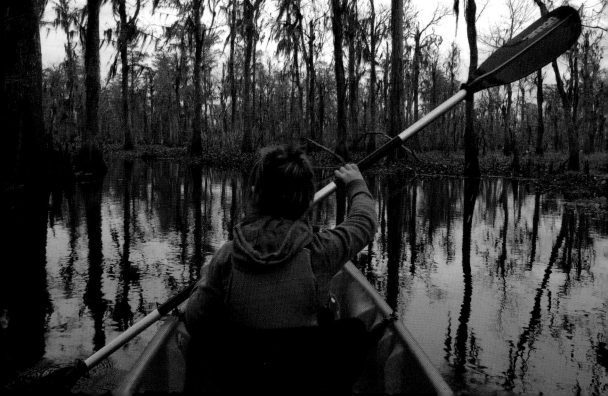

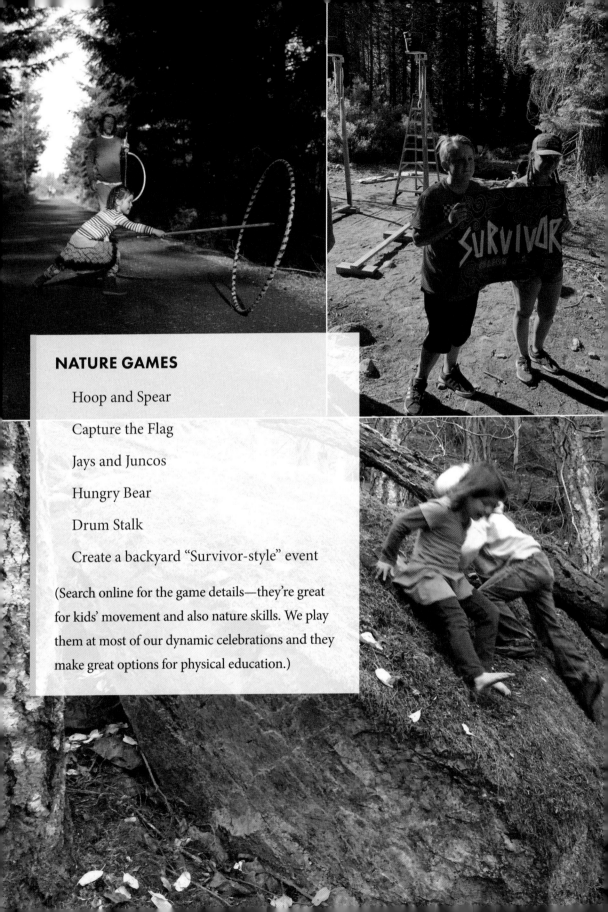

NATURE GAMES

Hoop and Spear

Capture the Flag

Jays and Juncos

Hungry Bear

Drum Stalk

Create a backyard "Survivor-style" event

(Search online for the game details—they're great
for kids' movement and also nature skills. We play
them at most of our dynamic celebrations and they
make great options for physical education.)

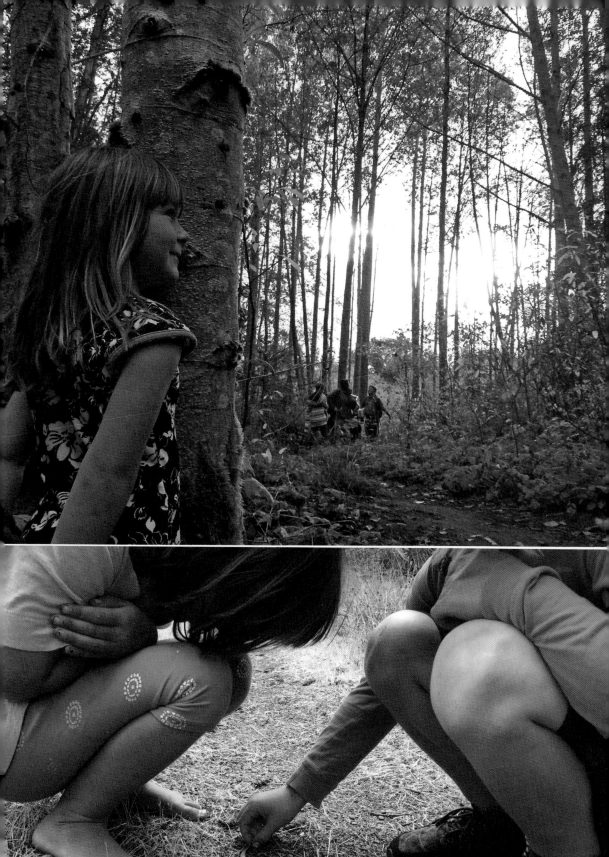

When it comes to movement and nature-rich activities, it might be helpful to find a teacher (for adults and kids) who has been through the hardening-off process and knows how to guide everyone through the outdoors safely. The world needs more people trained in educating or mentoring in this way, plus we need people advocating for public access to abundant green spaces. Could you be one of these people?

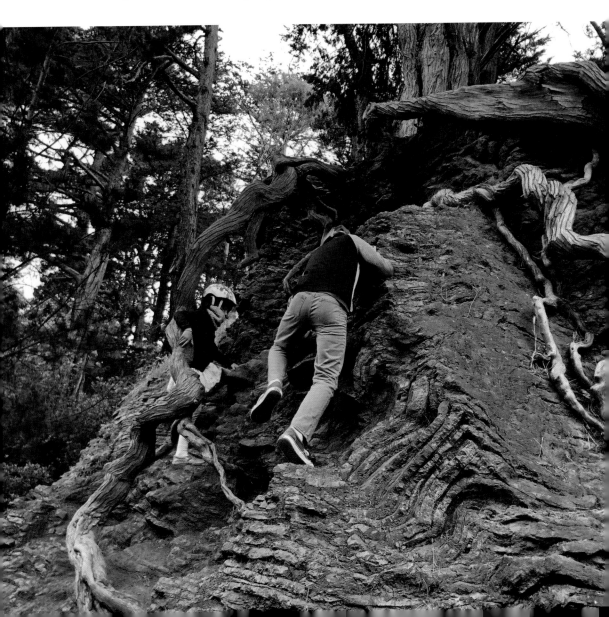

STUDY SESSION: SPORTS + SPECIALIZATION

Movement is like food. I SAID THAT ALREADY, I KNOW. But movement is like food. Eating a lot of a single food—even if it has nutrients—is not a well-balanced diet. Even eating a lot of a nutrient-dense superfood is not a balanced diet. We need to eat a wide range of dietary nutrients that cannot be found in even a handful of foods—and movement is the same. Kids' developing bodies need the opposite of specialization (getting good at one or two movements) when it comes to movement; just as dieticians encourage families to "eat the rainbow," kids need to be "moving the rainbow," so to speak.

There's a prevalent idea that if kids are going to be really good at a sport, they should start doing that one sport over and over again, starting as young as possible. Although there's a logic here, bodies simply aren't built for one narrow range of movement. They're built for a wide one, and it's this more robust "movement diet" that actually sets the stage for better sporting performance for older teens.

Many parents and kids might push towards specialization for sports success, even though most coaches and youth sports medicine boards advise against it. Each kid comes with their own passions, and if a kid "finds their flow" in a particular sport, you can motivate them to "eat more movement foods" by letting them know this will actually help their body perform better during their sport. Research confirms that being physically successful in more ways than one keeps repetitive use injuries down and supports the preferred sport in ways not currently understood. The ideal age to begin specializing is not clear, but current elite athletes seemed to have specialized between ages fourteen and fifteen; until then, a broad movement diet ultimately moves them in their preferred direction.

Jayanthi, N.A., E.G. Post, T.C. Laury, and P.D. Fabricant. "Health Consequences of Youth Sport Specialization." *Journal of Athletic Training*, October 1, 2019.

Kliethermes, S.A. et al. "Impact of Youth Sports Specialisation on Career and Task-Specific Athletic Performance: a Systematic Review Following the American Medical Society for Sports Medicine (AMSSM) Collaborative Research Network's 2019 Youth Early Sport Specialisation Summit." *British Journal of Sports Medicine*, February 3, 2020.

HOW DO DEVICES MOVE KID BODIES, EXACTLY?

While the walls and chairs of homes haven't changed much, today's kids are the first generation to grow up with such an abundance of in-home electronic media. Devices (televisions, computers, pads, and phones) each have different effects and these are different from the effects of what's being viewed; I consider devices effects on body shape and movement.

Just as we can categorize activities by the movement nutrients they provide, we can and should analyze what effect device use has on movement. For example, television viewing could be associated with sitting, but what if you're watching it while walking on a treadmill? Smartphone use could mean sitting and texting, or it could be playing an audiobook during a walk. The amount of time kids are spending outside is changing, but what they're doing when they're outside is also changing. A survey on "Children's Time Outdoors" in the *Journal of Park and Recreation Administration* (see Larson in this chapter's references) showed that in 2011 "being on media" took third place in reported "outdoor activities," after "hanging out" and "biking or running." Instead of playing tag, hide and seek, or a round of baseball in the park, kids are outside on devices. This is why we have to get specific about media consumption and all of its effects. What media are you talking about? How is it moving the eyes? The head? The shoulders? The hips? The bones? YOU GET THE IDEA. Perhaps one of the reasons we don't get specific is because we don't really want to know the answers. But without getting specific, it's too easy to miss critical information.

We are a group of humans that now have robust homes and, in many cases, numerous media devices for kids, including babies. When cigarettes first emerged they were everywhere and there was an *entire generation* that began smoking quite young. Several decades elapsed before a set of "use practices" was developed. Right now, parents and alloparents are the first generation to have to deal with raising children who are completely inundated with media devices. There is no framework offering guidance, likely because there is little understanding of this emerging (peaking?) problem. There are very few accepted good-use practices, and almost none of them relate to movement. As we put more devices in more places, and put more activities (education, entertainment, community) online, the baseline for "how much time is all right" keeps increasing. This is because the recommendations aren't trying to match our environments to our biology; they are matching them to our culture.

When kids started smoking cigarettes, I don't know if anyone said "well, cigarettes are here to stay, so we better get used to it." Regardless, it's still possible to understand what our human tendencies are and to figure out how to set up our environments and our good-use practices in a way that nourishes our bodies. We've done it before because we recognized we had to.

STUDY SESSION: WHEELS AND OTHER MOVES, TOO

Have you noticed that kids are growing wheels? Bikes, roller-blades, and skateboards are oldie moldies, but the list of wheeled movement is growing: rollerblades, hoverboards, Onewheels, scooters, and even shoes with embedded wheels are becoming the dominant movement environment for kids.

Wheeled movement is fast, stimulating, and involves its own set of skills, but it's worth contemplating how it moves kids' bodies. Consider specifically how this enjoyable activity, just like enjoyable foods, might make it harder for kids to develop a taste for slower-paced "movement foods" that pack more nutrition. While bicycling gets some parts moving and meets many of the categories of movement skills kids need (like balance and endurance), it doesn't move all of kids' parts, especially their hip bones, which need a lot of specific loading. Researchers have noted that only cycling throughout adolescence might negatively impact bone health. Again, it's not that cycling is harmful per se (I don't think cycling is harmful any more than a scoop of ice cream is), it's just not nutrient-dense enough to meet all the needs of a developing body.

Learning to ride a bike has become a rite of passage, but just as a culture might have a celebrated food, we don't want to confuse this "celebratory" food with an entire diet. Kids' bodies need other movements too.

My kids have bikes, scooters, and rollerblades, and they love them. We even started them young with strider-bikes (pedal-less bikes that cultivate balance skills long before kids learn to pedal), but we've always approached bike riding as dessert, establishing years of robust walking and other slower movement skills first. On a day-to-day basis, we also make sure our kids consume those baseline, necessary movement nutrients regularly in addition to any playful rolling.

Once kids are bike-formed, non-bike movements don't come as easily. Help them out and create the space for them to be able to do both well.

Olmedillas, H., A. González-Agüero, L. Moreno, J.A. Casajús, and G. Vicente-Rodríguez. "Bone Related Health Status in Adolescent Cyclists." PLOS ONE. *Public Library of Science*, September 30, 2011.

Rico, H., M. Revilla, E.R. Hernández, F. Gómez-Castresana, and L.F. Villa. "Bone Mineral Content and Body Composition in Postpubertal Cyclist Boys." *Bone*, 1993.

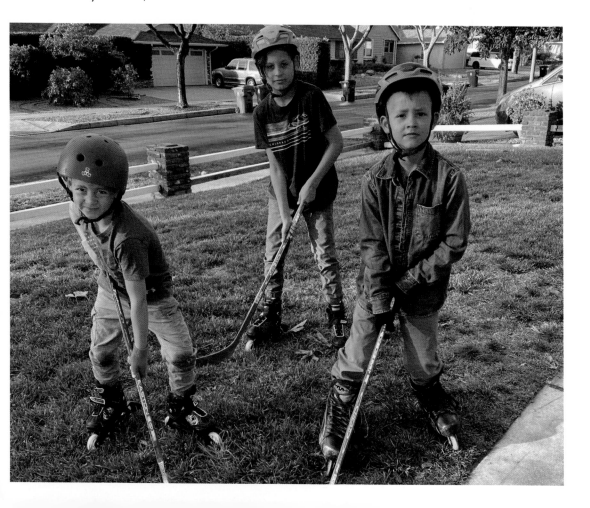

DO BABIES HAVE ACTIVITIES TOO?

The infant period of childhood is probably when children will be handled the most in their lives, but even so, our culture is relatively "hands off" when it comes to moving with our kids. Remember, bodies are always responding to their position, so we must ask, how are babies responding to spending so much time in repetitious, sedentary environments? You can look at babies as also having activities and see how their body parts are being moved. Where are they spending their time? In what environments? In what equipment? How is their body positioned or being moved? Our culture is hindered by the fact that babies are, in many cases, not being moved with a group of people (see: alloparents! Really, there's an entire chapter about them, chapter nine. You're almost there!). Babies need almost constant su-pervision. What a word! Super vision! They need our eyes and bodies to be on them constantly. Our culture has shifted in a way that means many adults no longer have time to provide this for their children, so in response we have created safe, still spaces to hold babies while our eyes (and arms) are elsewhere. These are cushioned places where they can't get hurt...but they can't move much, either.

I also dwell in a nuclear family a lot of the time, but my interests and training have led me to understand the essentialness of move-ment, so I had to get creative and make a new way for more move-ment when my babies came along.

As already discussed, being carried is a dynamic environment that moves babies a lot and is the time and place where they get to feel the weight of their head on their necks and backs. They respond by strengthening their torsos and spinal muscles. Now they have more autonomy to look around! If they're not given the strength to move their head, their curiosity-driven computers can only see a limited view of the world.

My husband and I decided this movement environment was the most important to us, and we used in-arm carrying almost exclusively. We didn't have a stroller and rarely used equipment other than our own bodies to hold or transport our babies. (As radical as that might sound, the bulk of the world does a combo of carrying and sling/ low-tech baby tie-ons. Our approach was like that, only with much less wearing and more carrying.)

The bonus stack here was that our bodies got super-strong. Baby-carrying is like a never-ending workout because they're always getting heavier; carrying them is a task that provides both of you with your movement needs. Pro tip: Work on good carrying alignment beforehand if possible, even doing more walking and in-arm carrying (groceries! library books!) before you need to carry a baby.

I had plenty of times where I needed to put the baby down! But babies come with their LEARN-MOVE-LEARN-MOVE software already running, and I needed to come up with ways to satisfy my babies' strong need to physically fulfill their curiosity. Some baby toys are designed to dangle above infants as they lie on their backs. These toys often play music or flash lights to keep some of their audience's senses stimulated, but I wanted to satisfy my babies' movement-hunger too. So I created my own setup for when I lay them down in order to have free arms for a while: baby chimes for punching. I knew my babies liked using their arms; their arms were always free when I held them, and they were already reaching forward. So our "punching chimes" were a set of cheap chimes that they could reach out and hit, practicing accuracy and getting a tactile and sound sensation at the same time. LEARN-MOVE-LEARN-MOVE.

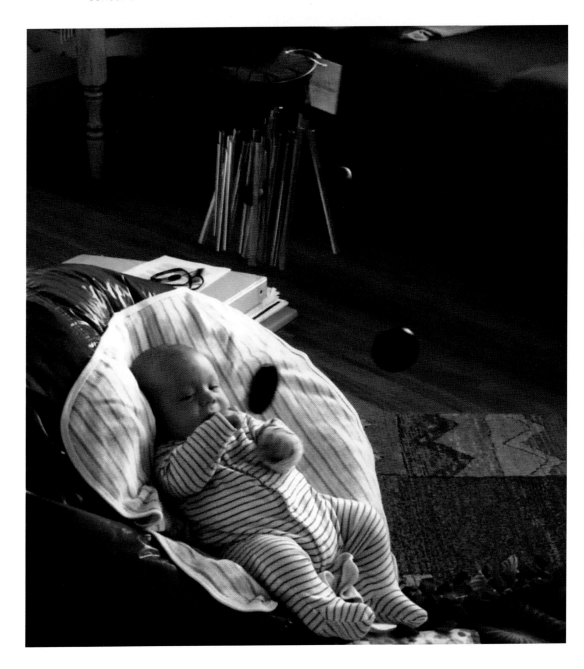

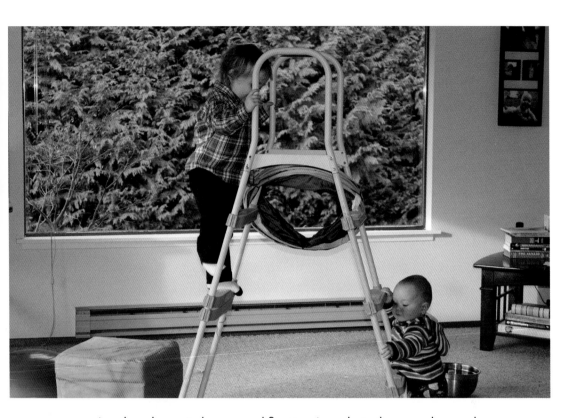

Another dynamic home modification I made in those early months was bringing in an above-ground pool ladder. This created a modified climbing environment that was stable, not too high, and could be approached stepwise. This was a must-supervise activity, but the ladder showed me how readymade even an infant's body is for climbing. Infants have movement reflexes—like stepping and grasping—that we fail to cultivate. They are often explained away as "vestigial" and no longer necessary, relics of when babies (and their community) used to have to move. But active babies show us these reflexes are still relevant and useful. They are hardwired, genetic catalysts for getting robust movement up and running right away. Human babies don't get up and move as early as baby deer or elephants do, but they can start to move earlier than we tend to set them up for. We can look to baby activities to support their movements and provide the environment that cultivates their LEARN-MOVE-LEARN-MOVE reflexes.

PSYCHOLOGICAL STRETCHING HOMEWORK

Being the one in charge of getting kids moving can be overwhelming, especially when we perceive change as taking a lot of work. Is it really worth it? Our bodies aren't the only thing we can exercise for greater mobility; our minds need practice to stay flexible. Diana Hill, PhD, is a psychologist and the co-author of ACT Daily Journal: Get Unstuck and Live Fully with Acceptance and Commitment Therapy. Below, she offers some homework adults can do to help break through psychological barriers to make the changes they'd like to.

Mental flexibility helps you stick with your desire to move more, even when difficult thoughts and feelings show up. Below is a set of exercises using "daily family walk" as an example. You can do this process for any of the move-more ideas you'd like to try from this book, e.g., "changing a living room setup," "cooking a meal outside," "writing a dynamic lesson plan," etc.

1. Get clear on your values

Values point you in the direction you want your life to head and they can re-energize you when your motivation wanes. Write out your top three reasons why taking a daily walk is important to you and put it somewhere you can see. Share the list with your family and have them write (or draw) one too.

2. Make a mini move

The best way to tackle overwhelm is to take your task and make it as small as possible. Small steps are more sustainable than big leaps. Start with a walk around the block. When that becomes routine, add on a tiny bit more.

Daily Family Walk
Values

1. I value getting the family off our devices at the same time!

2. I value body care and kids learning body care

3. I value spending time in nature

3. Welcome discomfort

Change is uncomfortable. Battling discomfort makes it worse. Practice willingness instead. Get curious. Is your resistance different before, during, and after a walk? Get open. Say to yourself, "This is what getting out the door feels like today!" Put out a welcome mat for chaos, disgruntled kids, and lagging energy and keep moving forward. The one guarantee is that whatever you are feeling, it will change!

4. Don't mind your mind

Sometimes our minds can be the worst coaches. Expect thoughts like "I don't want to" and "Dealing with my kids' protesting is too hard" or "We can walk later." You might not be able to turn off such thoughts, but think of them as an annoying jingle playing on the radio. They're just background noise and don't have to affect your plan.

5. Practice self-compassion

New habits are hard. Instead of being harsh or critical with yourself, offer yourself a kind, warm, encouraging voice. Remind yourself that starting something new like taking daily walks involves imperfection and missteps. When you are kind to yourself, especially when you get off track, you're more likely to stick with it, and you model compassion to your kids. Wouldn't we all be better off if we could be kinder to each other and ourselves?

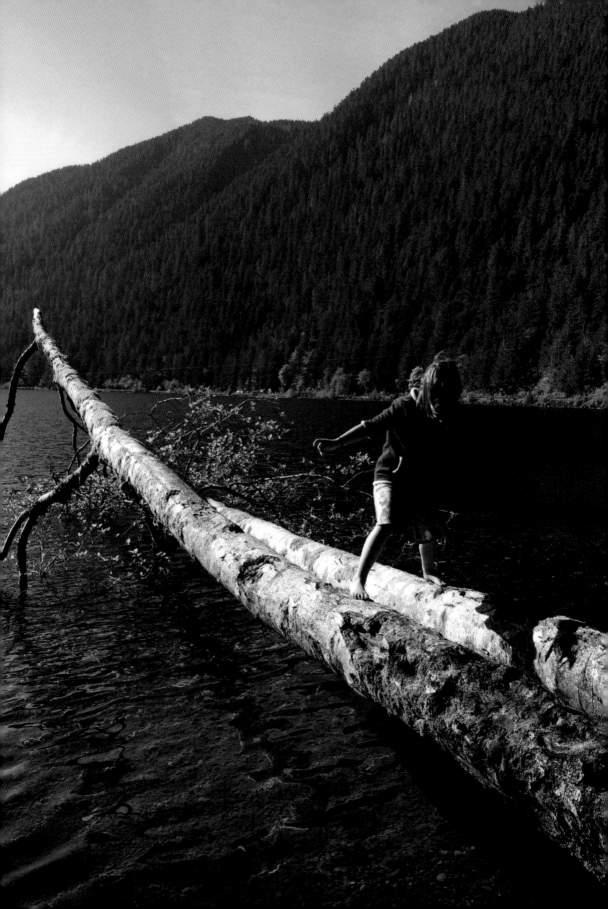

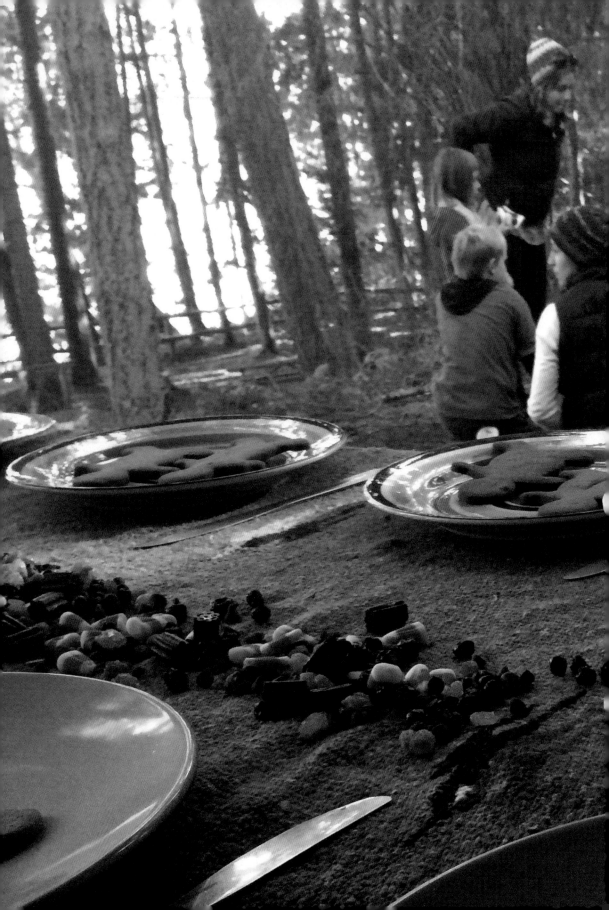

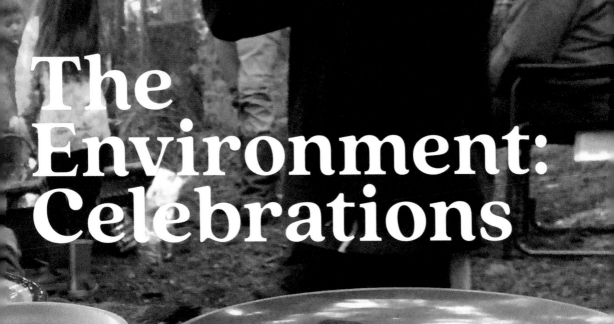

The Environment: Celebrations

Celebrating is marking an important event with the expression of our emotions via an activity.

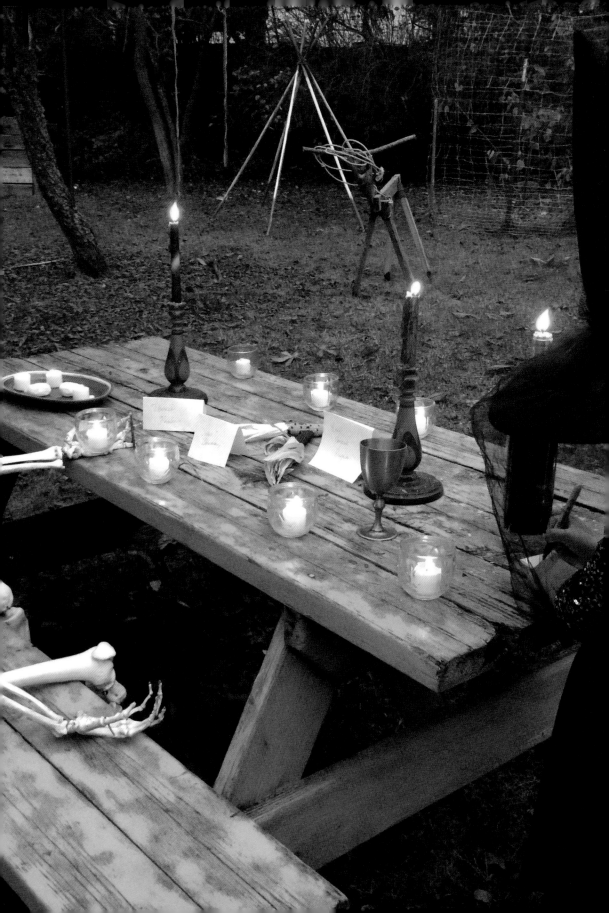

The Celebration Container

chapter eight

P op quiz! (Don't panic; you've got this.)

Q. How can we help kids get more movement during celebrations?

A. Hold celebrations outside

B. Choose a dynamic activity for the event

C. Have them do more of the "making" involved in party preparations

D. All of the above

Celebrations, like dwellings and clothing and learning, once involved much more movement than they do now. Celebrations used to be outside! In fact, the roots of most of our celebrations lie in natural occurrences like seasons.

In the pursuit of more movement and nature in all aspects of our lives, my family has been slowly converting our holidays back into the more nature-rich, movement-rich, community-rich events they once were. From décor-gathering walks to growing or sourcing special feast ingredients to organizing a friends-and-family hiking advent, celebrations are a time when many are keen to step away from day-to-day life, so why not make celebration time dynamic?

First off, *you can celebrate anything you want to*: the usual suspects, like holidays, weddings, birthdays, graduations, baby showers and christenings, death ceremonies, and also, "It's Tuesday," "First day of school!" and "It's been snowing for a week." Another thing about celebrating? You can do it outside—and simultaneously increase nature, people, and space in which to move. Just carrying the party-parts to the outdoors can move you more! Layer chairs with some blankets on the ground and you've offered a variety of sitting positions.

You don't have to wait for a formal celebration to come together; *coming together can be the celebration*. We regularly throw outside dinners—*for no reason*—in our own yard, in local parks, and at campsites (great options if you don't have your own outdoor space). And you do not have to do all the work! It is totally acceptable to have folks bring their own dishes or even their own meals. Simply initiating the outside gathering—sending a text with the date, time, location, and a note about how good it will feel to dine together outdoors—is often all the work you need to do to get your community moving together.

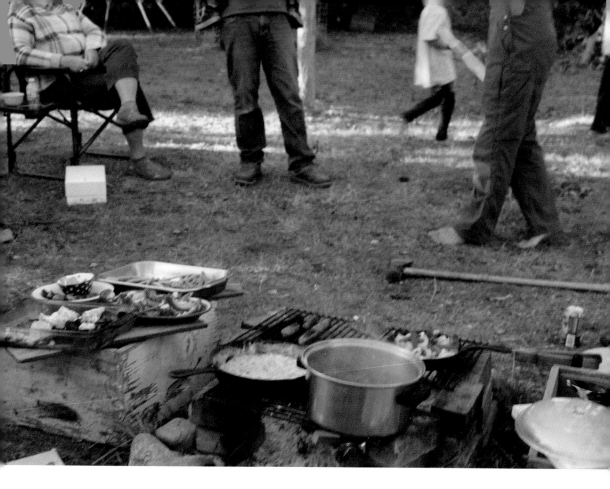

CHOOSE A DYNAMIC ACTIVITY FOR THE EVENT

Simple ways to increase the movement of a gathering include bringing out physical games—a jump rope, Frisbee, or Nerf guns—to create a little action on the side. Many celebrations include athletic activities or make them the feature event: swimming or roller-skating parties, a day barbecuing and playing at the beach, a game of football after a big family meal, a dance party that goes late into the night.

You can also host "food making" parties, where the making is the celebration itself. We've tried all sorts of SNACKTIVE CELEBRATIONS: gatherings where guests can try making things like butter (you don't need a butter churn, just cream and a jar), salt, maple-syrup candy (often last minute, because you never know when the trees' sap will start running) or contribute to harvesting crops, processing chickens, or making tamales!

These don't have to be huge offerings; they can take a few hours even on a

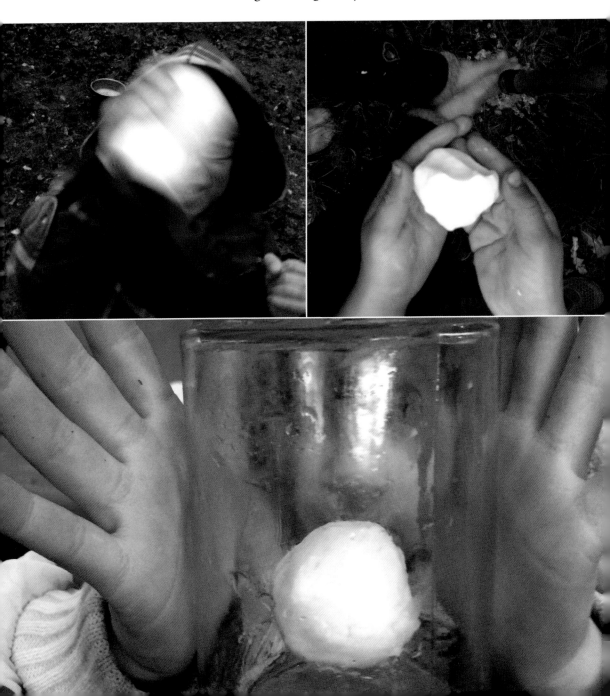

school night, and fill up after-school time with learning, dinner, and community, including time for a group of multi-aged kids to move together outside in less formal ways.

Not only can you move at a party, you can celebrate *on the move.*

Progressive neighborhood parties that travel from yard to yard are a great

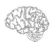 **MOVEMENT BIAS CHECK-IN: CELEBRATIONS**

As noted, nature is at the base of many of our celebrations, although many are unaware of these origins. Here are some questions to ponder that can help you find opportunities to move more.

- What does your family celebrate? Make a list. What is the role of children in these traditions?
- What is the history of your celebrations? What was the role of the children? Your elders?
- What were the features (e.g., foods or decorations) of these historical celebrations? What nature was involved? What movements?
- Make a list of the features associated with your celebrations today. How do they compare? What equivalents are you using? Where do they come from? What movements are involved?
- Do your children know the origins of their celebrations and your particular traditions? How much are they expected, allowed, or encouraged to participate? What knowledge of these traditions will they be able to teach to their children?

way to move and be nourished with your neighbors. We also created a hiking advent each year, trying to maximize the winter school break by moving outside together each day for a week. It takes little preparation beyond picking a short series of hikes that offer a variety of levels to meet our particular community's needs (e.g., paved trails for wheelchair access or places where it's easy for kids to participate for shorter lengths and then leave) and send out an invite.

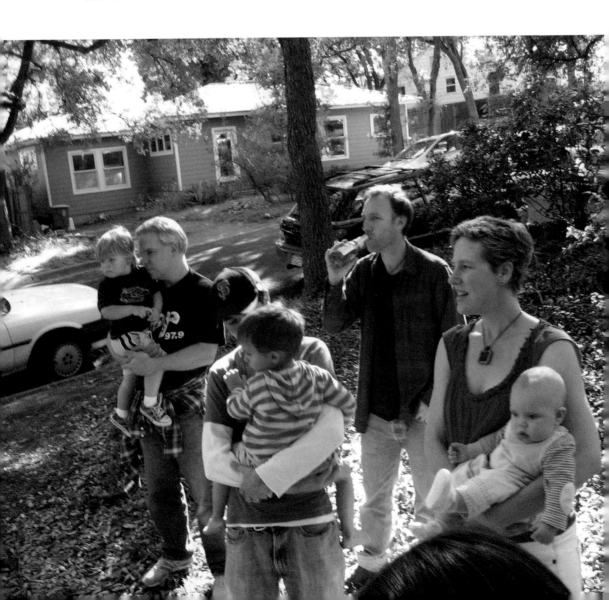

LET KIDS USE THEIR MAKING MUSCLES

I spent a childhood around adults who were stressing out, rushing around, feeling the pressure to make all the special things the holiday called for. The process didn't seem that enjoyable to them and it didn't feel enjoyable to me trying to keep myself out of the way. As an adult, I want to enjoy celebrations myself, so I get kids involved in preparing and making the celebratory elements.

Turn daily walks into "party walks" during which they explain their desired costume and how they're going to make it, or describe foods they'd like to have and how they might make them. Look for natural elements to gather on foot: items for table centerpieces, holly, wreaths, birthday bouquets, edible flowers.

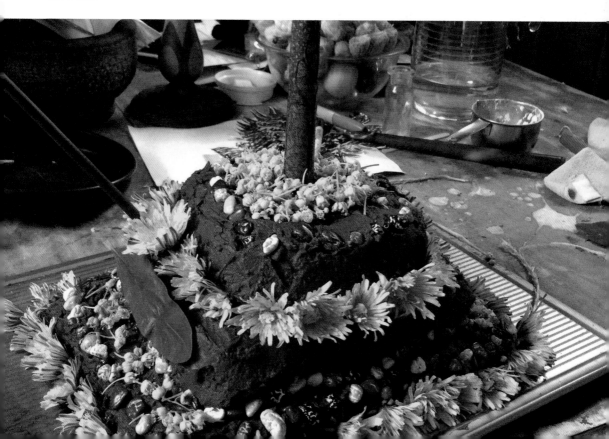

Walks to the grocery store to select special ingredients, hand processing spices (a great way to learn more about plants!), and even growing an essential celebratory item or two over the preceding months are ways you can stack celebrations *with all the other things.*

Kids can be in charge of party elements too! Kids can make the music, paint the faces, be the clowns, run the games, and lead the conga line. If we're trying to help children be in charge, and to "do" without needing it to look a certain way, what better place is there to practice than their own celebrations?

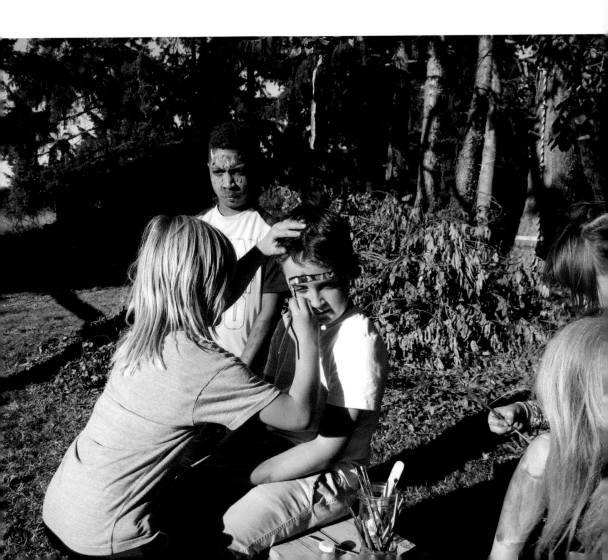

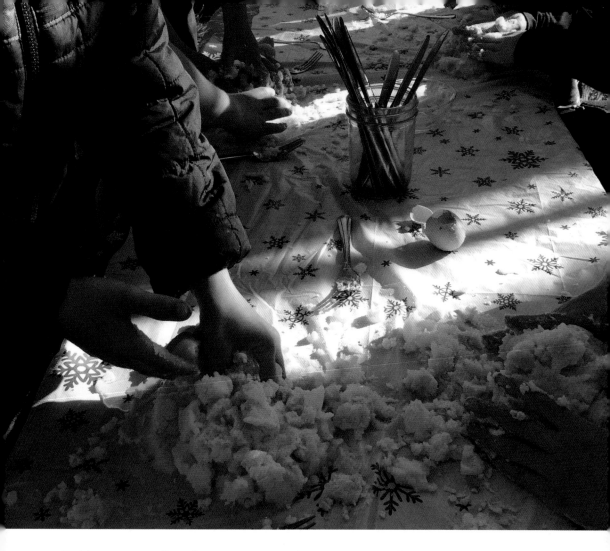

Moving more for what we eat can take extra time and prep work. I know that makes it challenging to fit into a regular day. Why not start with celebrations, then, where we've often set aside more time (or at least energy)?

We had a kid who wanted pesto gnocchi pasta for their birthday meal, so what better time to figure out how to make it? I had some things prepared to save time, and set up a big kids' table outside where they each mixed their own batch of dough, then rolled and cut out their pieces before bringing them to the water to cook them.

These food and outdoor moves weren't the focus of the party—it was a birthday celebration—but they still ended up being the star of the party, perhaps due to how rarely kids are now offered "hands-on" activities of such importance. They were in charge of making the celebratory meal, yo!

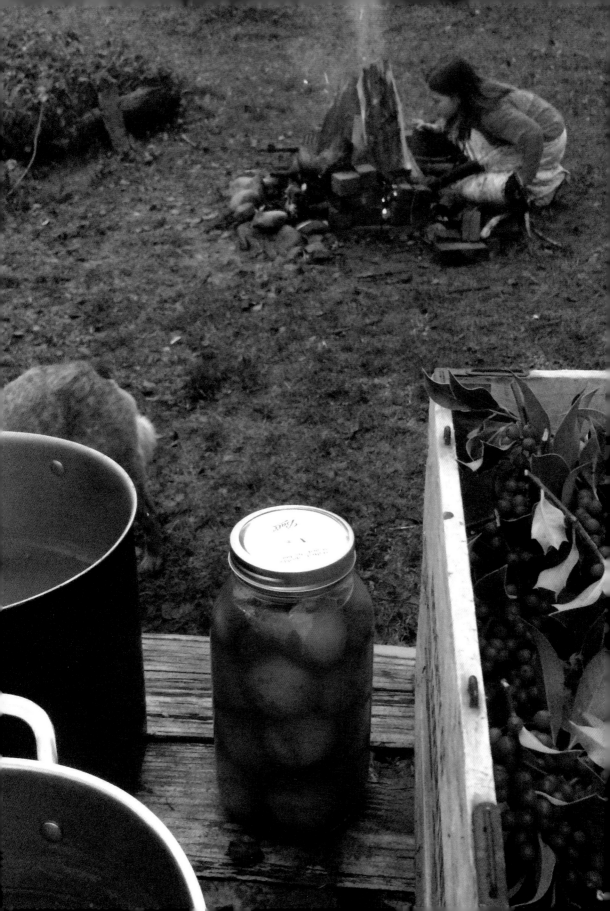

Solstice Celebration Recipe (modify as needed)

- ONE TEXT: "Friends, meet at our house to fill a mug with cider to sip on a group night walk to celebrate the dark, then back to the house for a yule log and fire for cooking. Bring your own mug and whatever you'd like to roast."
- ONE PRE-EVENT HIKE to gather (50 bundles of holly)
- ONE FIRE for pre-walk warming, snacking, post-walk warming and ceremony
- TWO POTS of apple cider (donated by one of the families), mulled
- FOUR LADLES so folks can dip their own
- ONE JAR of homemade plum-infused brandy (because #spirits!)
- FOUR HOURS of outside winter time
- TWO HOURS of group walking
- ZERO HOURS of house cleaning, before or after, because it's an outside party
- mix
- inhale
- repeat next year

Like all recipes, you can adapt this to your celebrations, community needs, and landscape, but the core of it remains. It's also important to note that celebrations don't require you provide all things at all times. My offering, in this case, was the space and the invitation to join me for things I was going to do anyway. "Bring your own food and cups to the party" is a perfectly acceptable invitation if it gets folks to gather, celebrate, and move more often. Try it and see.

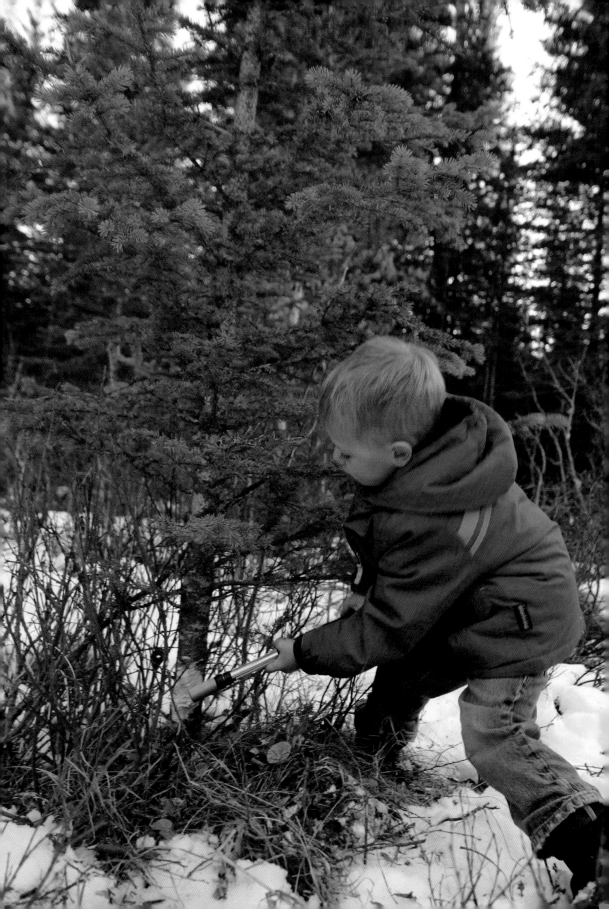

CREATE YOUR OWN CELEBRATIONS

Researching and engaging with our own cultural traditions has been informative and healing for my family, but traditions are also dynamic and limitless. For that reason I like to create additional traditions, formal and informal, that get us moving. One example is birthday walks.

Our family celebrates birthdays, and our yearly rite of passage for our kids is their "birthday walk." This is where we take a family walk that's as long as our child's new age. We use miles, but it could be kilometers or blocks or whatever you choose! While we're walking mile one, we tell one-year-old stories, and on mile two, two-year-old stories, etc. This doesn't have to be on

SHOW AND TELL

A great way we get our kids to move more is to create family traditions that require it. One of our favorites is our Halloween costume hike; our kids dress up in their costumes and we let them loose in the forest. There is magic in pretending to be a bumblebee or a fire-breathing dragon in the woods. We also go on a leprechaun hunt for St. Paddy's Day, cut down our own Christmas tree, create Valentines with nature materials collected on a family walk, and clean up as much trash as possible in our neighborhood (specifically on Earth Day, but on every walk too).

— Rosanna Taylor

their actual birthday (although sometimes it is), but rather how we create a metaphorical journey to celebrate the one they've made around the sun. Sometimes the kids bring a friend or two, and sometimes there are surprises along the way, including others that join in partway or show up to celebrate as we move.

Even when celebrating older traditions, tweaking them to meet your needs is allowed. Ask yourself how they can be tweaked, then ask your kids and wider communities.

This book is about getting more movement, but there's a deeper payoff for everyone, including kids, when you increase your movement via a "stack your life" approach. When we move more for what we use in our celebrations, we end up making the celebration longer and fuller! Movement extends and deepens our rituals. It can restore them. To celebrate is to mark an important event by expressing our feelings—joy, grief, reverence, gratitude, anticipation—via some activity. Celebration is an active process. The more movement, the more celebration (more learning, more community, etc.). GET IT? Who doesn't want more celebration in their lives?

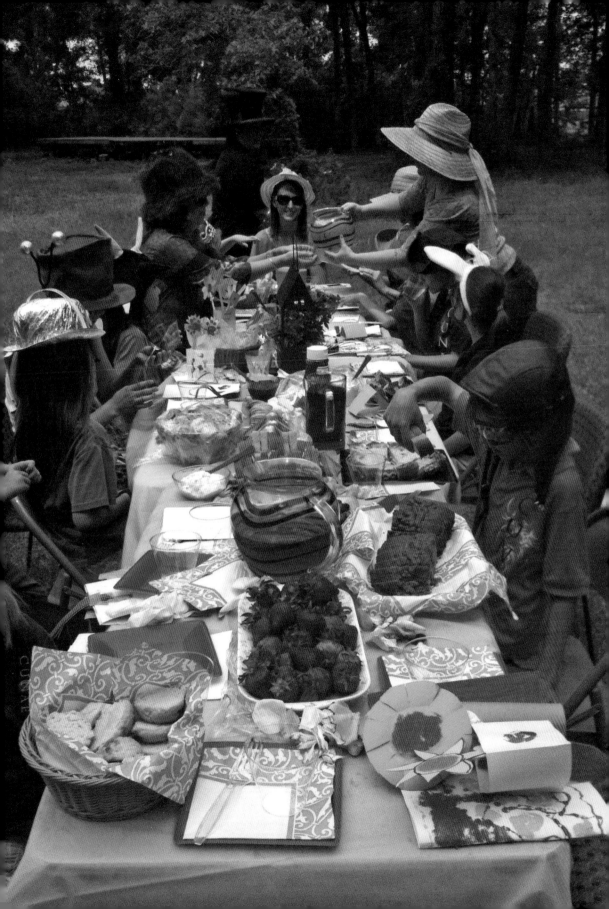

DYNAMIC GRIEF

Grief is a natural reaction to loss. The grieving process lives inside the NATURE circle, but it also lives inside the CULTURE circle. Traditional grieving practices often include abundant vocal and dancing movements of the entire family and also the entire community! Like many of the other celebrations discussed in this chapter, death ceremonies have become sedentary. What is the role of movement in the mourning process, and how does the lack of it in death ceremonies and mourning periods affect children who are grieving?

Wild Grief is an organization striving to create a vital, resilient, and connected community with a healthy response to death, one that makes space for grieving youth by cultivating their presence, connection, and a sense of belonging with the earth. Learn more at wildgrief.org and on Instagram @wildgrief_olympia.

Young children's grief doesn't look like sitting in a circle answering a facilitator's questions. When their grief is touched, sometimes they climb over the couch, grab their sibling and roll on them, move around the room, or throw their bodies on the ground. All of us experience grief in our bodies, but for children, movement is the primary way grief is expressed.

The founders of Wild Grief had all experienced the death of an important person in our lives, and we'd all been volunteering to support kids and families who were grieving, which is where we met. Independently, we each had a deep connection to nature that was a very important part of our lives. In the volunteer work we were doing with the support groups and the camps for grieving kids, we noticed

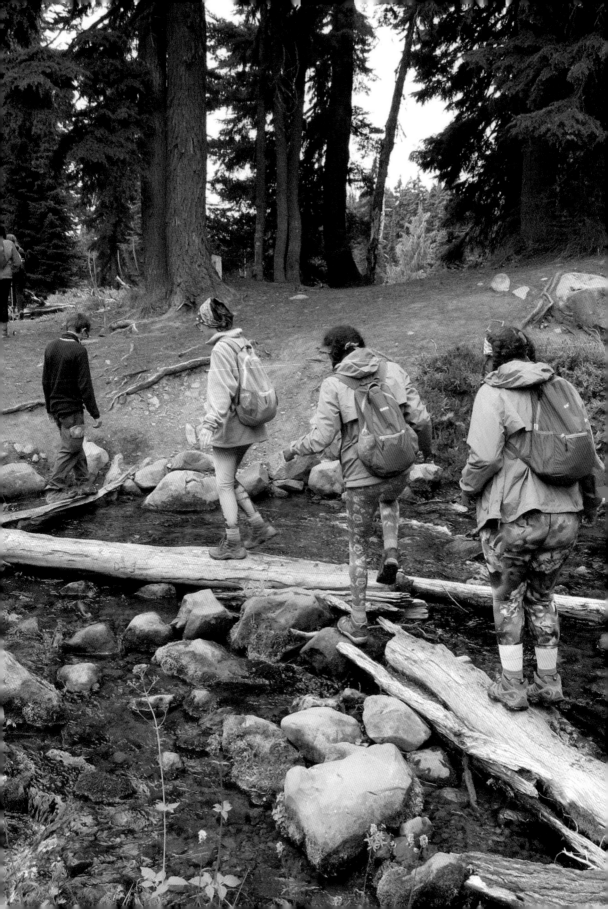

that the times where those kids were outdoors, their grief work really took on a new dimension. It was more transformational. We wanted to spend more time and attention on that aspect of being outdoors and depending on your body to move you place to place and take care of yourself, which made it easier to support grieving teens. It can be very challenging to convince a group of teens to come sit in a room and talk with strangers about grief and hard stuff. Instead, an experience where they're going backpacking, they're learning a skill, they're being outdoors, takes a little of that pressure off and gives them a lot more space to be able to share what they want and what they need to when they're ready.

Talking is a part of the process, but it's not the only part, and can be limited. Grief is an embodied experience that we move with, not only speak about. To learn and to make meaning, we need to have some physical, multisensory experience, a personal emotional connection, and movement to really integrate our learning. Grief is the ultimate experience of learning who you are, what your mortality is, what it means to have someone close to you die—there's so much learning and integrating that kids need to do. Trying to do that only in our brains doesn't really work.

Wild Grief offers programs for kids, teens, and families who have lost a loved one: hikes and backpacking trips as well as virtual programs with independent experiential activities and nature connection. Hikes open with a sharing circle where participants can share about their grief experience, and always include periods of walking in silence, giving each person an opportunity to enter into a relationship with the environment, to land in their bodies and on the earth. Some stay in silence, and some move into small group conversations where they talk about everything from their really intense grief experience to what else they're doing that weekend. There's no right or wrong way, but the hike is a chance to acknowledge we're here together, talking about our grief, walking through our grief.

On our backpacking trips, we're creating a physical experience that matches some of the grieving process. The first day of the hike the theme is "grief is hard." Grief can hurt and it can be discouraging, just as the first day on the trails can be, as participants are heading uphill, maybe on their very first backpacking experience, carrying this heavy pack and trying to figure out what it means to sleep outside. Making these links between the physical experience and what it can feel like to be in grief really opens up a lot more avenues to explore what grief is and how to normalize it.

The natural world gives to us as we move through it. It engages our curiosity, draws our attention to details, transmits a sense of peace, a healthy regard for danger, offers us metaphors, invigorates our breathing, or takes our breath away. By changing the pace, it allows us to hear the little whispers that are ignored in our busy lives. Moving through a complex natural environment gives our grief arms and legs, eyes and ears to feel, process, and integrate.

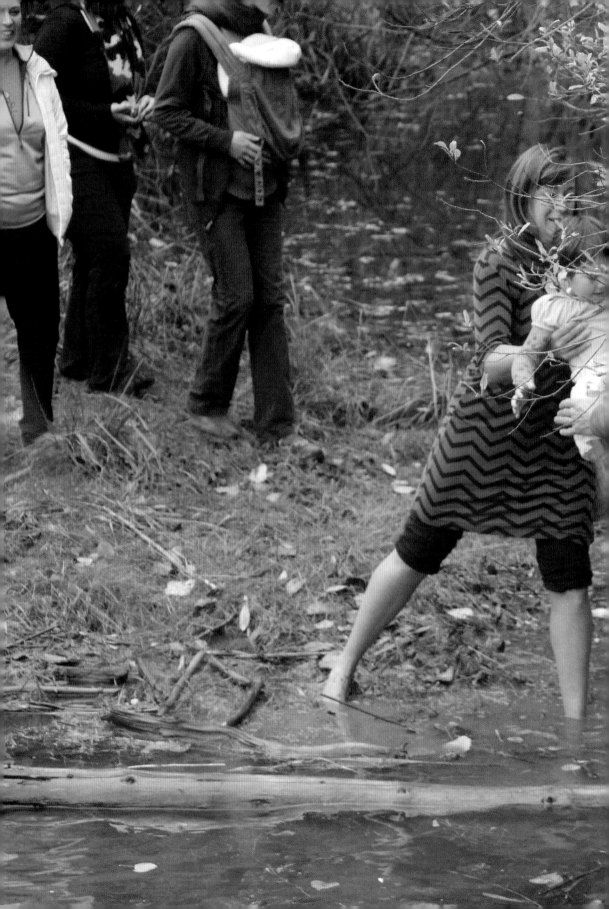

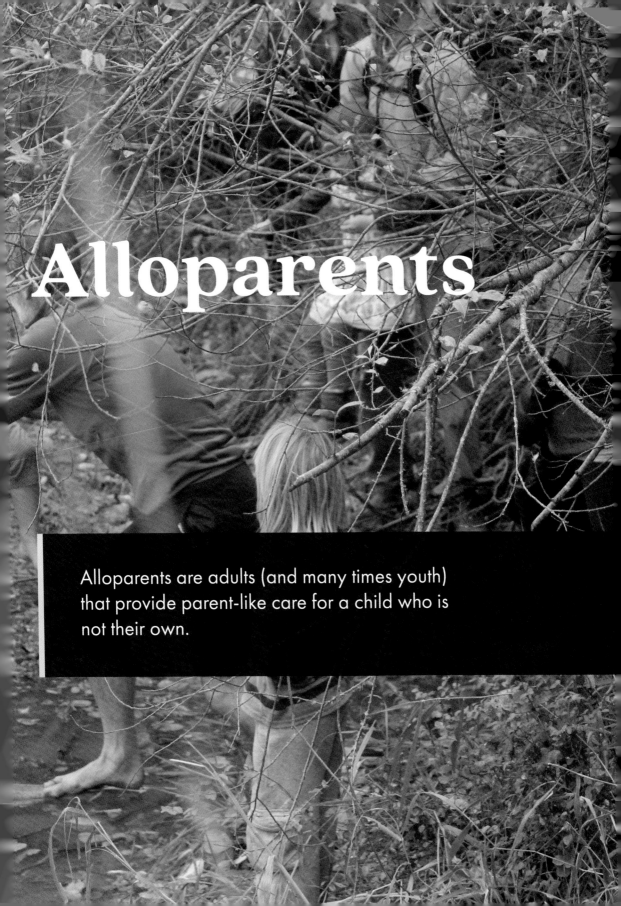

Alloparents

Alloparents are adults (and many times youth) that provide parent-like care for a child who is not their own.

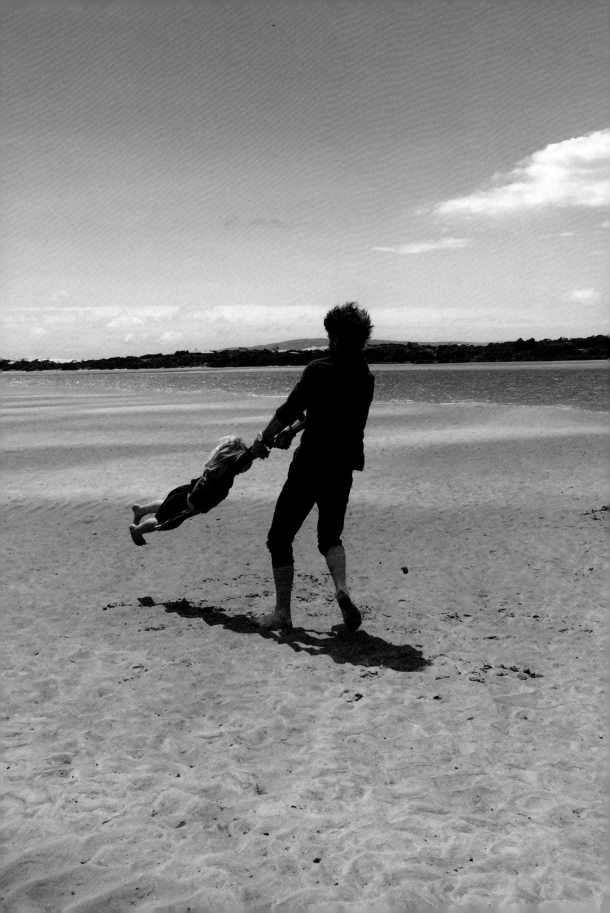

Alloparents

C hildhood takes a long time. I already said that, right? Well, it does, especially from a child's perspective. But you know who else often laments that kids require a lot of care for a long time? Parents. It is said that the days are long and the years are short, and I know that when I'm older I will be wishing I could go back to my younger years of more intense parenting, but today (and next Thursday, too) I could use a big fat break.

Humans have long childhoods and knowledge-heavy diets, but the success of both depends on another human feature: *other people*. When we list the features of a natural environment, which is the environment our bodies are wired for, we include things like trees and bugs and birds and bacteria and hard, lumpy ground. But do you know what else needs to be on that list of "things in nature children's bodies are used to moving through?" A group of other people who care greatly about them. Not only in the general sense (I care about everyone!), but in the direct, personal sense. Human children and their parents need others who are tangible and help to provide direct care.

If intensive childcare over a long time sounds fatiguing, that's because it is. This is why the "anatomy" of a group of humans includes *alloparents*: people who provide non-parental childrearing support. Humans come from a variety of landscapes that each have their own physical features. Similarly, who allocares and how they allocare varies by group. Still, the universal element is that people other than parents care for children.

THE WHOS AND HOWS OF ALLOPARENTING

Today, we are not very far from a traditional parenting setup. Parents still share the work to raise children; alloparenting just looks different. Of course, there are still close friends and family members (aunties and uncles, siblings, grandparents) who participate in a child's life and relieve parents, but now the list of alloparents also regularly includes daycare workers, teachers, coaches, and healthcare workers. There is also a new alloparent in town: portable screens that deliver captivating content on demand are a brand new way to keep kids occupied and safe (which most often translates to "still") so the adults can tend to other needs.

In addition, alloparenting arrangements are now far more formal than in the past when everyone lived in close societies. Parents could once step out to meet their needs while children folded seamlessly into a group that wasn't immediate family but still felt like it. By definition, being alloparented should feel no different to the child than being parented, and in this way, today's alloparenting is much different—not only in the who, but the how.

Although there are absolutely wonderful teachers in school (and I and my kids have had so many of them!), it's easy to imagine the overall difference in warmth and acceptance at school compared to the warmth and acceptance

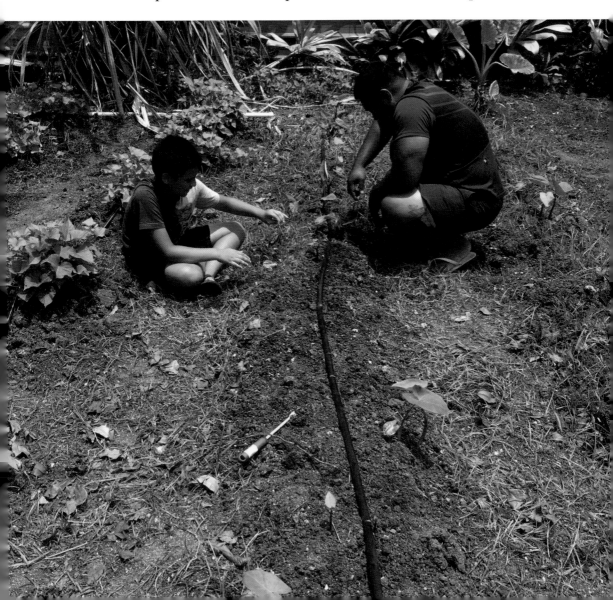

you'd receive if your uncles and aunties were your teachers. The new adult-to-child ratio alone changes up the amount of direct and personal care.

Another part of the *how* factor is what is being transmitted during that time. Traditional alloparenting includes more than offering a place to stay safe within while the parent is gone; an alloparent's role has included furthering the knowledge children will need to be successful.

Although candy can turn off hunger signals because it's high in stimulating, sugar-rich calories, candy offers no other nutrient. Similarly, many alloparenting environments kids are spending their time in are meeting fewer and fewer of their needs. Kids are kept out of immediate harm, just as candy can keep kids alive compared to not having anything to eat, but what about all of those things they still need from alloparental input but aren't getting?

When alloparenting becomes low in interaction—between other kids, between adults and kids, between children and the diverse input of the natural world—but high in stimulation (videos! candy!), can we even continue to call it alloparenting? I think we can, in the same way we still call it "soil" even if all of the nutrients have been depleted. Still, we need to regenerate these growing grounds for children. Alloparents need to stack it, and add back in the movement, learning, nature, rest, etc. that children depend on getting from their community.

All of this is to say that we still have an alloparenting system, it's just one that matches our sedentary, industrial landscape.

Whether alloparental care is done in a more formal institution of daily care, such as education, or it's provided by family (or chosen-family) allo-parents, the alloparental system we use today is a sedentary one because our whole culture is sedentary. We still use a complex social network to share the raising of our children…only nobody's moving.

CHILDREN (AND THEIR PARENTS) NEED MORE OTHERS

I said before that children need others, but that's only half of the story. Children and their parents today are *surrounded by others,* but the others aren't helping, and they can often make it harder.

Why do humans alloparent? For multiple reasons. Babies come with "I'm suuuuper cute, don't you want to hold me?" technology that beckons the young and old alike. But also, the way we respond hormonally to babies is based on exposure. It could be that being around babies and children throughout a lifetime tunes our biology into better meeting their needs. We might be an alloparenting group because being raised in an environment of alloparents has shaped our bodies to be able to do this job. Finally, we might be sharing the work of those parenting because we ourselves will need help in the future—maybe with our own kids, or with our own care once we're an elder. And who will be there to help you other than those *you* helped? So, by being alloparents, we're able to meet our needs to give and receive love (and touch and movement) beyond any parenting years we might have, but if that's not motivating, alloparenting is also how we invest our energy into the

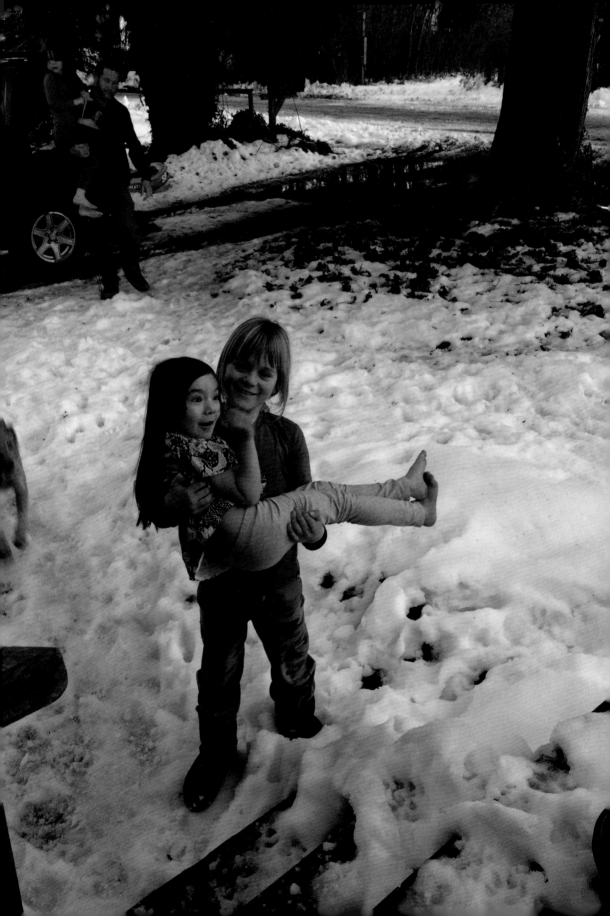

big bank of "please take care of me later," which you will certainly be cashing out at some point.

A side effect of the way we have institutionalized and outsourced "help," from childcare to eldercare, is that we have effectively gotten rid of the environment that developed and kept our alloparenting muscles in shape naturally.

In smaller communities that still have the more traditional "who" and "how" intact, everyone gets daily, hands-on experience with kids (including kids who are not their own). In contrast, today's culture leaves many people entirely unpracticed in the very natural phenomenon of caring for children. If our arms and their million-year-old climbing technologies can't develop the ability to hang from a branch in today's landscape, then certainly people who have not grown up with children at every age and stage can wind up entirely unpracticed at using the "muscle" of considering and caring for them or their needs.

But here's the deal: while we might be inside our houses and out of that tiny circle of green spaces we call "NATURE," we're right in the middle of that giant-circle-that-is-everything, NATURE. The rules are the same. Who makes up these entities—professionals, governments, and other organizations—that will care for us in the future? GROWN-UP CHILDREN. So again, we're right back where we started. We should all contribute to our young generation because they're the ones who end up caring for us, if not directly, then through the work they're able to do.

We are all alloparents; we've simply lost this awareness because we're not moving through environments that would have naturally clued us in. We've put all the "kids and kid people" into their place and non-kid people into another. But because all of our actions affect the people around us—including kids—we're all always influencing kids, whether we mean to or not, by being and creating their cultural container. Our lack of awareness when it comes to what kids need (in this case movement) doesn't change the fact that we all create environments, make rules, set expectations, and act as examples in everything we do.

Right now, the world needs more dynamic alloparents. It needs leaders, teachers, and supporters of nature schools. It needs movement teachers and programs dedicated to keeping children active and robust. It needs dynamic babysitters and daycares, and grown-ups willing to gather neighborhood kids and walk them on an adventure. It needs more folks who can communicate with children and understand their particular needs. Don't get me wrong; parents can do these jobs too, but parents have already taken on a great deal of work when it comes to children. The world needs those who aren't already doing so to invest time (and let's be honest, their brain cells and other once-useful body tissues) into the children who will eventually support them, either directly or by paying tax.

A culture is made up of children, parents, alloparents, and their beliefs and their behaviors. If you want to make the culture more dynamic, then move. If you're moving more, you're demonstrating to kids how to move more. If you're walking and playing in your neighborhood more, you're mak-

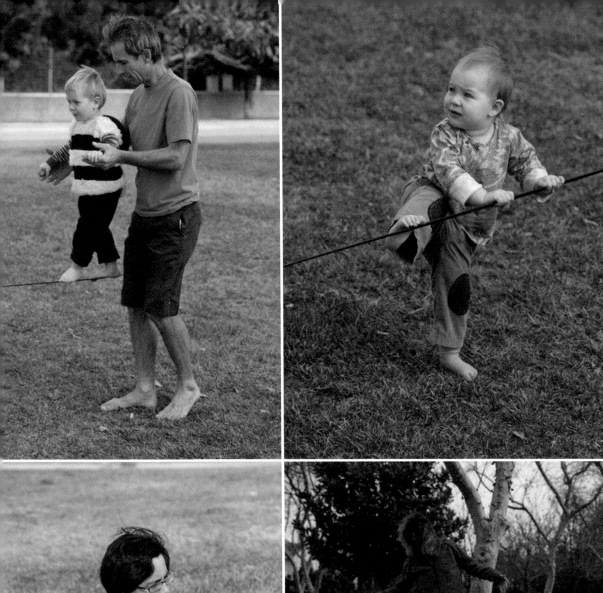
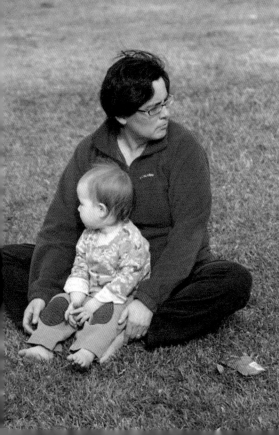
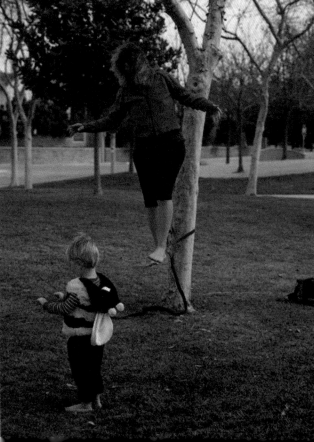

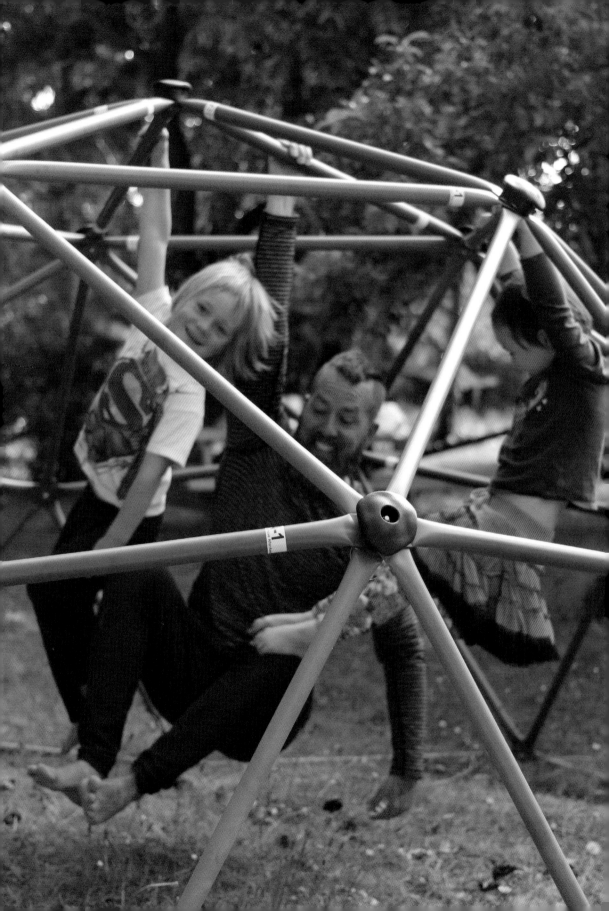

BIAS CHECK-IN: ALLOPARENTS

The exercises below can help parents and alloparents alike assess beliefs they hold about their roles as well as any deeper thoughts on parenting and alloparenting.

- Make a list of all alloparents who have supported your child, and in what way. If you're a non-parent, make a list of the ways you have supported a child/children.
- Make a list of the additional support you and your child could use when it comes to movement (or accomplishing any of the ideas in this book). Be specific; what exact support would help? Non-parents, what skillsets do you have or are you interested in developing that would support a movement-rich, nature-rich life for a child? Be specific; what do you need to make these happen?
- Make a list of your own caregivers when you were growing up, including the landscapes/non-human elements. What did each provide? What lasting effects did they have on you?
- Consider these statements and note what thoughts, feelings, or sensations arise:

  "I don't really like any kids but my own."

  "I'm no good with kids."

  "I have no experience with kids and don't know how to talk to them."

  "It is not appropriate to bring children to this restaurant/wedding/airplane."

  "You can't travel with children (or ought not)."

  "Nobody can care for a child like a parent."

  "Nobody will care for my child as well as I will."

ing that area safer for others to also move through. Set up a slackline. Start cartwheeling. Race off to a tree. These aren't just movements, but an invitation—an invitation to the culture (and its children) to move.

CREATING A DYNAMIC COMMUNITY

A more common word for what alloparents provide is "community." Humans have always been in nature and have always been in nature with a community of others. Community is an element of nature, but its importance is so great that we've teased it out as something separate. And it is distinct; nature is like a multivitamin with numerous necessary compounds, one of which is community. After all, we can go into a forest alone and meet some of our needs, or we can go with our immediate family and meet even more needs. Or

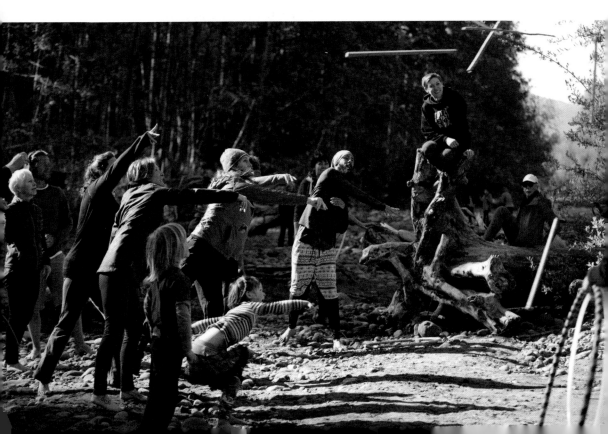

we can go with a more diverse community that is made up of individual needs but focused on a collective goal. It is the latter that produces the richest, most rewarding experience.

I've found "Vitamin Community" to be such a simple way to stack. Take the thing you were already going to do and ADD OTHER PEOPLE. Adding community immediately makes a task more nourishing, and suddenly— magically—it is easier to get everyone moving more. Community is people carrying your baby because they adore her, and long group walks. Community is teachers and hunting guides. Community is group soup nights, a meet-up at the barbecues in the local park, and the person sharing their front yard with the neighborhood. Community is elders with time, lost knowledge, and patience for endless questions. Community is adults who don't have children but love playing with them or teaching them. Community is children just slightly older than yours, beckoning them to catch up; it's children who are younger and eager to be led. Community is others knowing the children in your group and seeing them for who they are and what they need.

There are many types of communities that involve children: sports or school-centric, faith-based, cultural, arts-related. Kids likely already have a community or two. The question is, can they become more dynamic? Can meetings move outside or on foot, can celebratory events involve more hands-on activities (getting more little hands moving), or can movement simply be put on the agenda? After all, every tradition has movement at its roots!

SHOW AND TELL

Living in a rural environment, we are Destination Grandma and Grandpa. With the luxury of what we call the deep woods, I wanted to cultivate areas that call to the grandkids. One of those places is the snack cave. I located an area on the property where the natural environment provides a cave-like atmosphere. After a long day of clearing, it was ready.

The kids are at an age where the journey is a big part of the adventure, so we never take a direct route to the snack cave. There

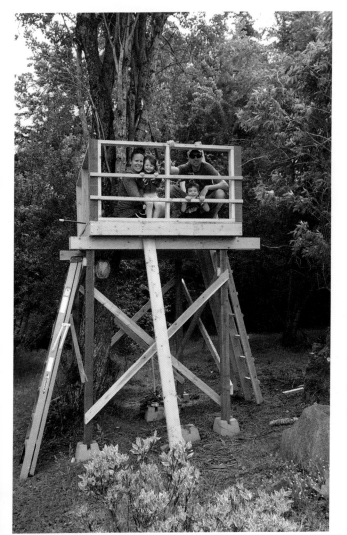

are plenty of opportunities to wander around, over, and under everything the deep woods offer. The family, including our five-year-old grandson, also built a tree house with two different ways to access it. There's nothing like climbing up into it to eat dinner! Having things like shovels, and even bananas to feed the neighboring cows (who knew that cows love bananas?), available when they visit invites exploration. And exploration always invites movement!

—Cindy Hurlbert

SHOW AND TELL

How can I consistently get more vitamin "N" into my life and those of my two young daughters, spend more time with friends, and move off-road more? I sent out a group text to a few of my friends with kids letting them know that I would be starting an after school hiking club and just like that, "Wild Wednesday" was born! The group varies from week to week in number, age, and level of "wild." As a rule the kids lead the hike. They run up and down the path often detouring for no set amount of time in the mini ravine. Occasionally we briefly talk about the plants that surround us. We've snacked on wild wood sorrel (lemony and kid approved), identified poison ivy, and even slayed a few bags-full of invasive weeds. Every week I look forward to meeting a new group of wild and free spirits on the trail and soaking up all their energy and excitement for the little things in life all while getting my much needed tree therapy. It's a beautiful hour in the middle of the week!

— Jessica Kennett

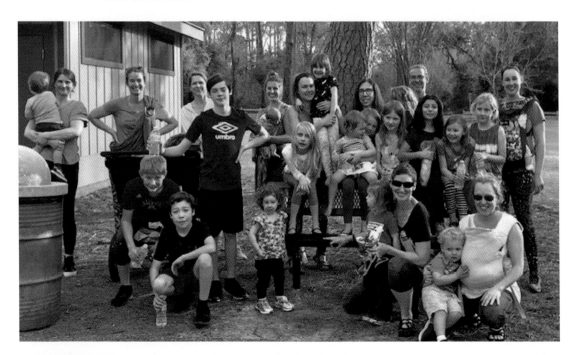

Another approach is to create a community that *centers* around movement. Children are in a similar boat to adults—a boat that is stuck in the sand, unmoving. Parents and alloparents are unsure how to launch it, and everyone is frustrated. So start something! A Saturday morning group walk, a park barbecue, a field-game day, a backyard clothing swap, a community garden. Pick up some extra kids on your next hike. Walk over an invite. Send a text. These are the humble beginnings of community.

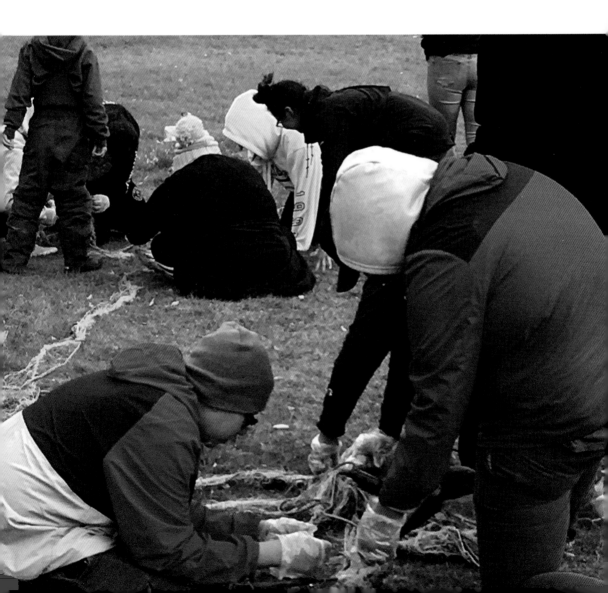

RECOGNIZING *ALL* OF THE ALLOPARENTS

It's no big surprise that compared to cultures that don't see themselves as separate from nature, our culture recognizes the care provided by humans more than it recognizes the contributions of the non-human elements of nature. The *other* others.

Remember the forest? That forest is alloparenting the entire village.

"The village" is made up of human children, parents, and alloparents. But who else protects, nourishes, and teaches these humans? The forest. The forest offers them protection. It provides them with nourishment. And with these gifts, the forest can teach people about successful, ongoing relationships.

Our society uses non-human entities to contribute to children's development (screens). Likewise, many traditional cultures celebrate the contribution made by non-human and non-living entities of their landscape. They appreciate those entities greatly and grant them greater equality than we do. If screens can occupy a child, then so can a pile of rocks, or a flock of birds in a tree, or storm clouds rolling in. The processes are the same, but the medium and the knowledge kids step away with are different.

Our society is trying to get kids and adults moving, and it's also trying, desperately, to save forests—but right now the direct relationship between all of these isn't clear to us. When humans can no longer successfully move in and around trees, when humans can no longer successfully move outside, the essentialness and perceived value of trees and their landscape quickly diminishes. "Going outside" and what's out there comes to be viewed as dangerous. We've made trees a hindrance. We can no longer climb trees. We can no longer *see* any trees, and we definitely cannot see the forest. Our giant greenhouses are blocking the view.

This raises a classic debate about what determines why children are the way they are: do their genes, *by nature,* pre-program them to "come this way," or are they a blank slate that is shaped by how they're cared for, or *nurtured,* once they arrive?

I've always felt that the answer is "both, of course," or as Andrew Solomon writes in *Far From the Tree: Parents, Children and the Search for Identity,* "nature *via* nurture."

To add to the already complex relationship between genes and nurture, I ask: what happens to children when the way they're nurtured is nature-free? What happens to humans? If the physical elements of green-spaces nature provide care, knowledge, and the physical robustness necessary to better live alongside them, then we must move the discussion forward. We must consider *nature via nurture via nature.*

What I've come to understand is that I have few parenting "skills" and even fewer tricks. Did I remember to tell you at the beginning that this is *not* a parenting book? WELL, IT ISN'T. When it comes to parenting, I open my heart, put down my head, and literally step through whatever that day holds for me. My approach is this one-note song I sing to my kids: everything is better when we go outside together and move. Let your alloparents—the trees, the birds, the weather, the tracks—tell you a story, make you a costume, feed you, and fill you up. Let me learn, adorn, and eat alongside you, for these are my alloparents, too.

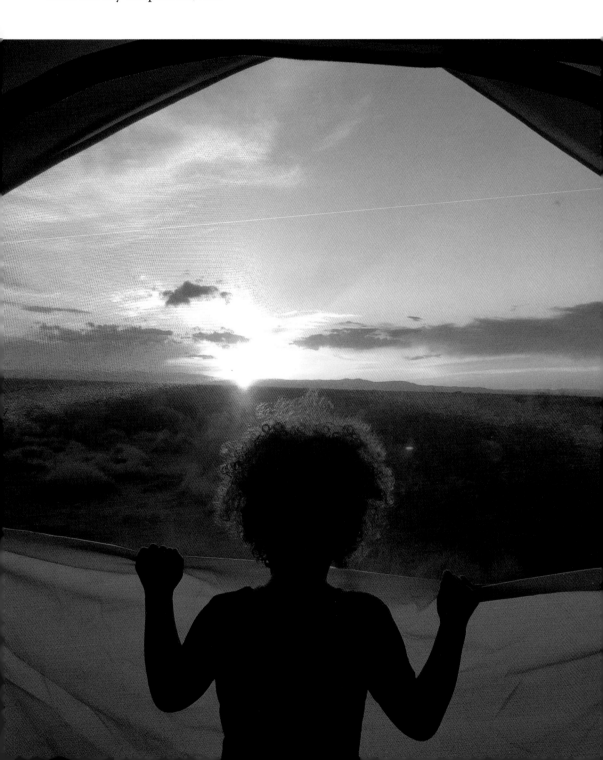

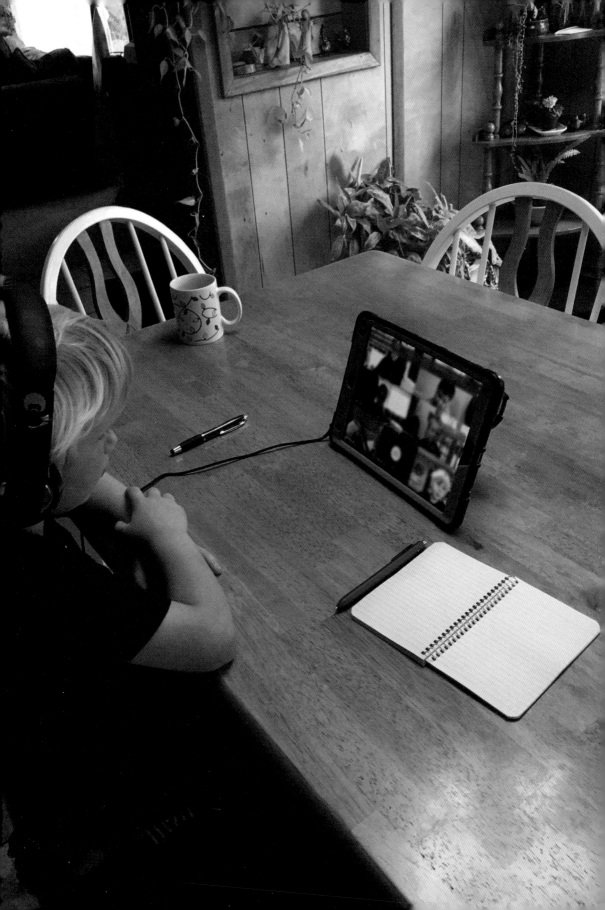

Afterword

Grow *Wild* has been in the works for years, but it is coming out amidst a pandemic that began to emerge in 2019—a pandemic that serves as a reminder that we do, in fact, live inside an environment larger than culture: we live in and are a part of nature, and nature is not always benign.

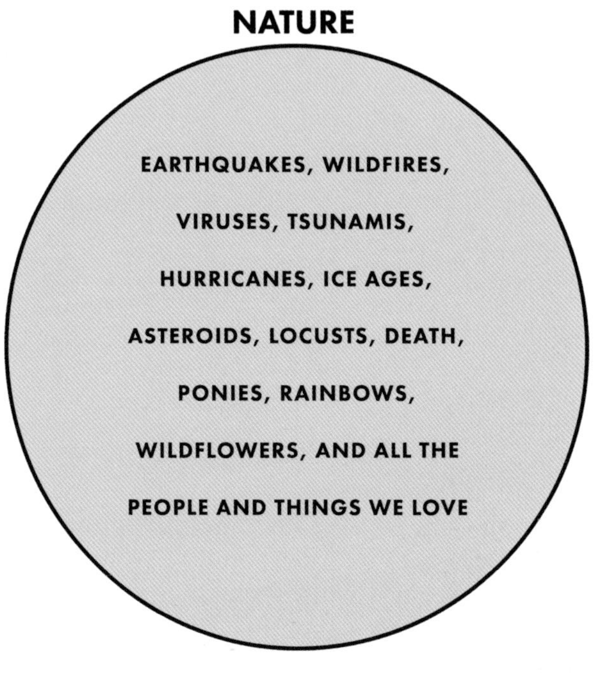

NATURE

EARTHQUAKES, WILDFIRES,

VIRUSES, TSUNAMIS,

HURRICANES, ICE AGES,

ASTEROIDS, LOCUSTS, DEATH,

PONIES, RAINBOWS,

WILDFLOWERS, AND ALL THE

PEOPLE AND THINGS WE LOVE

The intersection of the COVID-19 pandemic and *Grow Wild* was not lost on me. One of the reasons I advocate for maximizing our movement to our personal capacities—especially in the form of more purposeful movement on the individual level—is because the infrastructure of the technologies that stand in for our movement play a role in how viruses can emerge. Not only can the sedentarism that comes with hyperconsumption increase the rate of virus emergence, our lack of individual movement can make us more susceptible to the effects of many viruses. A large group of people not moving can place humanity as a whole in an extremely vulnerable position.

While writing, I knew many of the practical ideas in this book might be labeled "throwback," "retro," or even "quaint." Some people might even consider them outright outdated. This is often the logical conclusion for someone who has lived a life in which they've done almost none of the labor necessary to keep them alive; someone who hasn't gone looking to see how and by whom that work is done.

The irony is that our very tendency to perceive certain movements as unnecessary requires that other folks, including children, do the movement for our benefit. Adults and children walk miles to squat and search through dirt and water looking for minerals like coltan that our "move less" portable electronic devices require. They tend to and harvest plants, bend for hours to pick fruits and nuts, gather and process plants for oil, process things by hand. Many of these workers are enslaved; see the U.S. Department of Labor's report in the afterword's reference section for a list of the products that come from such conditions.

Laborers have most often formed the backbone of "civilized groups," and our current sedentary culture is only possible because 1) we're benefiting from the movement being done by others and 2) we regularly use a massive set of technologies that move us or deal with the side effects of not moving—an exoskeleton, so to speak—which we, like a hermit crab, use for our protection.

Even if all of our necessary items are eventually produced by a worldwide army of machines and all the world's knowledge is accessible to everyone on a portable device, machines are still made of things that come from the earth that will need to be harvested and powered by a harvest. Even if we are able to achieve "sedentary parity," where there are no humans relegated to gathering something from the earth via physical labor powered by food and sun, the massive built infrastructure and energetic needs to sustain such a system would have to envelop the planet while still falling short of supporting our lifestyles.

That all being said, without having to move more deeply into the sci-fi plot already emerging, right here (earth), right now (today), moving one's own body over the earth to extract things from it is not outdated—it's completely current. Our survival still depends on these movements being done, including movements to produce food and clothing; we're just not the ones doing them.

Movement is counterculture, and this implies that being sedentary is the norm. But normal doesn't mean optimal: despite being countercul-ture, moving more is a wise choice, the benefits of moving more exist, and research supports the choice to move more. Whether or not something is mainstream or counterculture is merely a numbers game. If most people don't move but you do, you're now behaving *counter* to the bulk of the crowd. Being counterculture can feel like you're on the incorrect or wrong path (or certain-ly the less traveled one), and that's often what keeps us from changing. But I'll just remind you: a large mass of people behaving in a particular way says *nothing about the validity of that behavior*, only that there's a large population doing it.

One paradox of a sedentary culture is its ability to hyperconsume. While it seems like massive numbers of people not moving their individual body parts with any great frequency wouldn't be able to extract many resourc-es from the planet, the opposite is true. The sedentariness of many people demands that other people farm, mine, and otherwise extract in areas where humans haven't spent much time before.

This is how new viruses can emerge. As humans begin to interact with other animals—wild ones as well as those they domesticate or raise in new environments—they can be exposed to viruses those animals carry quite benignly. Like humans, viruses seek to grow in numbers and their ability to repeatedly mutate themselves allows them to occasionally infect new species.

There have always been viruses, but it takes a large group of humans to create an epidemic and an even larger, well-connected group to create a pandemic. As the novel coronavirus emerged and began to capitalize on our population size and connectedness, its ability to spread rapidly was somewhat slowed by how quickly humans can now spread information around the globe. This created a habit-altering situation on a global scale never experienced before in our time. Almost overnight, we reduced our already waning physical movement when many people sheltered in place to slow the spread of the coronavirus. This also reduced our interaction with other nutrients: nature and community.

Research into early COVID-19 effects on children's movement found significant decreases in physical activity, especially in older kids, and significant increases in sedentary behavior (as well as time spent on a screen). Kids' physical activity had already shifted from traditional unstructured free-play to predominantly organized activities and sports. When sports, clubs, and gym class were cancelled, kids were simply unaware of or unpracticed in other ways of moving, and in some parts of the world they weren't allowed to go outside to play. Their sedentary behavior took the form of video, television, movie watching, playing computer and video games, and sitting for schoolwork. In one sample it was noted that only ninety minutes of daily sitting were associated with schoolwork; the other eight hours of sitting were for leisure-time activities.

But not all movement was lost. While there was a decrease in overall physical activity, kids who weren't confined indoors started taking walks and using their neighborhood areas for movement. Traffic was down, making it possible to move near our homes again (just let *that* unintended consequence of a car-centric culture sink in). Researchers point out that city planners could make streets safer for walking as a way to promote kids' physical activity *during the pandemic*—but why stop there? The fact that children are unable to walk and move where they live is a problem that should demand immediate attention, pandemic or not. Some areas have made changes, and decision-makers should consider making them permanent to meet the movement needs of all citizens, including kids.

Many folks also turned to "heritage pursuits"—those seemingly vintage practices like making bread and sewing with their families. Gardens began popping up for a variety of reasons: educational purposes, food security, a dose of outdoors, or simply to fill the time. While kids' steps-per-day might have fallen to the basement and their minutes on a screen crashed through the roof, there was also a natural shift afoot toward many of the solutions outlined in this book. Why? It could be that these activities were lurking under the surface all along, waiting to emerge when we had the time or home spaces. Perhaps some people, for the first time, saw the fragility of many of the systems we've come to depend on and started to take action.

The pandemic has provided a pregnant pause. Pregnancy is often a time of change. Not only in the obvious physical way, but in the hyper-thoughtful consideration we give to our choices and behavior during this time. For many, pregnancy is the first time they deeply consider personal nutrition and rest, which are necessary movements to keep the body intact or prepare it for the marathon to come (and by *marathon* I don't only mean the labor of birthing; I'm referring to labor needed for a lifetime of child-raising behavior). Pregnancy naturally creates more energy, often directed to cleaning and organizing our space into something more suited to what's on the way. Pregnancy is a time of heightened awareness not only for the pregnant person, but for everyone involved. There is often a whole community of people holding a deep desire for the newest "other person" to succeed.

Similarly, the pandemic has created a shift in consciousness for many of us; a time where a culture is pregnant with the possibility of choice: how will we move forward now that we've seen how radically different our lives can look? Many children's movement activities have moved online. Will this remain, creating more screen time (and demand for more devices) for us all going forward? The pandemic has created a widespread use of the word *essential* when it comes to some types of work. What does *essential* mean in this case? Why are so many people doing non-essential work? Why are so many not working for their own essentials?

Humanity is currently considering how to solve many social and ecological problems, yet we never discuss how our cultural sedentarism relates to these issues. I propose that moving more can contribute to solving some of them.

Future pandemics are one such problem: viruses will continue to jump to abundant new hosts, and virologists warn that our continued hyperconsumption and its associated environmental impact will see new viruses emerge at a greater rate than in the past.

What I love most about moving more in a stacked way is that its beneficial byproducts are also stacked: greater physical resiliency, less consumption, and less waste. Some folks pursue a "minimal" life by reducing their belongings directly; I've found that pursuing a movement-rich life achieves the same outcome indirectly. If your intention is to maximize purposeful movement, you often need to get stuff out of the way to make that happen. The intent is to meet your needs maximally; the minimalism is simply a side effect.

We talk about the future with terms like "carbon footprint" and "climate change," but this language divorces the problem from our individual behaviors. If I'm not stepping, then carbon is. Carbon's footprint is where our own footprints once were. That move-less exoskeleton "greenhouse" our children are now born into *emits gases*. Gases that go on to create a global-sized greenhouse (is everything wilting a little now?), making it difficult for anyone or anything to step outside the effects of a sedentary culture. GREENHOUSE GASES. Get it?

If we perceive that these terms relate more to the global economy, industry, and nations than they do to us on the individual level, the solutions appear to require great technological advances—the expansion of our "greenhouse" or exoskeleton in which we want to take shelter like the hermit crabs—rather than stepping back or stepping up the work that's still required by our bodies. If we can stay grounded in what technologies represent at the most foundational level (i.e., stand-ins for our personal movement), it keeps the baseline from moving.

We can adopt more solar and wind power, but we also have abundant *human* power at our fingertips, a "technology" already built in—and that power is renewable! Moving is how your body becomes able to move more; our fuels are food and sun. We've been searching for "greener" ways to fuel the industrialized systems that a culture's ability to be sedentary depends on: massive amounts of pocket-sized information, transportation, medicine, caretaking of children and elders, education, agriculture, and entertainment—instead of how to reduce the burden of the systems themselves. Many depend on these systems for their life, and many depend on them for their ease. As humans equally wired to move and to capitalize on all opportunities *not* to move, it's likely that we are biased—by our very nature—against seeing the bigger picture.

But it is not just the planet that is paying the price for our sedentarism. Millions of dollars go into research and buildings, machines and gear designed to get people exercising because human sedentarism has never been so abundant, and the numerous and costly health risks associated with being sedentary are well established. Despite the data and the urgency, movement is still declining. At the research, clinical, and government levels, people rarely talk about movement outside of exercise—even though we know by now that relegating movement to a single hour a day is a) a fine start but not enough movement and b) still more time than many people have to spend on something that doesn't meet any other needs for them or their family. We can all move more, in a well-balanced way, when movement is made more relevant to our lives rather than to merely our health—which is already something many have learned to sacrifice in exchange for participating in this type of society.

You can move more with kids because you can meet more of everyone's needs; you can move with them more because you're interested in the physical and emotional benefits. You can move more with kids because doing so places less burden on other humans, human societies, and the non-human elements of the world. You can move more simply because it's fun.

Whatever your reasons for moving more, your movement matters. *Our* movement matters. Our movement matters to the forests and the trees, the village and the villagers. Movement matters to humanity's children.

REFERENCES AND RESOURCES

This is a list of references, noted resources, as well as additional reading that has shaped the ideas in *Grow Wild*, even if they were not called out specifically. You can find this list online and linked at nutritiousmovement.com/growwildresources/. "Study Session" references are in their respective sidebars; all others are organized by chapter below.

Entire books that have informed my overall perspective presented in *Grow Wild* or make for great continued reading include:

Hewlett, B.S., and M.E. Lamb. *Hunter-Gatherer Childhoods: Evolutionary, Developmental & Cultural Perspectives.* New Brunswick, NJ: Aldine Transaction, 2009.

Hrdy, S.B. *Mothers and Others: the Evolutionary Origins of Mutual Understanding.* Cambridge, MA: Belknap Press of Harvard University Press, 2011.

Mann, C.C. *The Wizard and the Prophet: Two Remarkable Scientists and Their Dueling Visions to Shape Tomorrow's World.* New York, NY: Vintage Books, 2019.

The Children & Nature Network hosts a large, curated database of peer-reviewed scientific literature making the case for children's need for nature: https://research.childrenandnature.org/research-library/

Introduction

American Friends of Tel Aviv University. "First Evidence of Farming in Mideast 23,000 Years Ago." *ScienceDaily,* July 22, 2015. https://www.sciencedaily.com/releases/2015/07/150722144709.htm

Anderson, L.B., J. Mota, and L.D. Pietro. "Update on the Global Pandemic of Physical Inactivity." *The Lancet,* September 24, 2016. https://doi.org/10.1016/s0140-6736(16)30960-6

Garner, L., F.A. Langton, and T. Björkman. "Commercial Adaptation of Mechanical Stimulation for the Control of Transplant Growth." *Acta Horticulturae,* 1997. https://doi.org/10.17660/ActaHortic.1997.435.21

Guthold, R., G.A. Stevens, L.M. Riley, and F.C. Bull. "Worldwide Trends in Insufficient Physical Activity from 2001 to 2016: a Pooled Analysis of 358 Population-Based Surveys with 1.9 Million Participants." *The Lancet,* September 4, 2018. https://doi.org/10.1016/S2214-109X(18)30357-7

Hall, G., D.R. Laddu, S.A. Phillips, C.J. Lavie, and R. Arena. "A Tale of Two Pandemics: How Will COVID-19 and Global Trends in Physical Inactivity and Sedentary Behavior Affect One Another?" *Progress in Cardiovascular Diseases*, April 8, 2020. https://dx.doi.org/10.1016%2Fj.pcad.2020.04.005

Kohl, H.W., C.L. Criag, E.V. Lambert, S. Inoue, J.R. Alkandari, G. Leetongin, and S Kahlmeier. "The Pandemic of Physical Inactivity: Global Action for Public Health." *Lancet Physical Activity Series Working Group*, January 18, 2012. https://doi.org/10.1016/s0140-6736(12)60898-8

Lamoureux, N.R., J.S. Fitzgerald, K.I. Norton, T. Sabato, M.S. Tremblay , and G.R. Tomkinson. "Temporal Trends in the Cardiorespiratory Fitness of 2,525,827 Adults Between 1967 and 2016: A Systematic Review." *Sports Medicine*, November 3, 2018. https://doi.org/10.1007/s40279-018-1017-y

Song, C., H. Ikei, and Y. Miyazaki. "Physiological Effects of Nature Therapy: A Review of the Research in Japan." *International Journal of Environmental Research and Public Health*, August 3, 2016. https://dx.doi.org/10.3390%2Fijerph13080781

Chapter 1: Stack Your Life

Bowman, K. "Move Your DNA: Movement Ecology and the Difference Between Exercise and Movement." *Journal of Evolution and Health*, 2017. https://doi.org/10.15310/2334-3591.1077

Harris, A.R., P. Jreij, and D.A. Fletcher. "Mechanotransduction by the Actin Cytoskeleton: Converting Mechanical Stimuli into Biochemical Signals." *Annual Review of Biophysics,* May 2018. https://doi.org/10.1146/annurev-biophys-070816-033547

Hartig, T., R. Mitchell, S. de Vries, and H. Frumkin. "Nature and Health." *Annual Review of Public Health*, January 2, 2014. https://doi.org/10.1146/annurev-publhealth-032013-182443

Khan, K.M., and A. Scott. "Mechanotherapy: How Physical Therapists' Prescription of Exercise Promotes Tissue Repair." *British Journal of Sports Medicine*, April 14, 2009. http://dx.doi.org/10.1136/bjsm.2008.054239

Kuhn, S.L., D.A. Raichlen, and A.E. Clark. "What Moves Us? How Mobility and Movement Are at the Center of Human Evolution." *Evolutionary Anthropology*, June 17, 2016. https://doi.org/10.1002/evan.21480

Chapter 3: The Clothing Container

Ashdown, S.P. "Improving Body Movement Comfort in Apparel." *Improving Comfort in Clothing*, March 27, 2014. https://doi.org/10.1533/9780857090645.2.278

Carroll, K., M. Alexander, and V. Spencer. "Exercise Clothing for Children in a Weight-Management Program: Semantic Scholar." *Journal of Family & Consumer Sciences*, January 2007. https://www.researchgate.net/publication/234728446_Exercise_Clothing_for_Children_in_a_Weight-Management_Program

Théveniau, N., M. P. Boisgontier, S. Varieras, and I. Olivier. "The Effects of Clothes on Independent Walking in Toddlers." *Gait & Posture*. Elsevier, September 4, 2013. https://doi.org/10.1016/j.gaitpost.2013.08.031

Chapter 4: The Cooking Container

Angier, N. "Why Childhood Lasts, and Lasts and Lasts." *New York Times*, July 2, 2002. https://www.nytimes.com/2002/07/02/science/why-childhood-lasts-and-lasts-and-lasts.html

Bird, D.W., and R.B. Bird. "Children on the Reef." *Human Nature*. Springer-Verlag, June 2002. https://doi.org/10.1007/s12110-002-1010-9

Bird, R.B., and D. Bird. "Constraints of Knowing or Constraints of Growing?" *Human Nature*. Springer, June 2002. https://doi.org/10.1007/s12110-002-1009-2

Giudice, M.D. "Middle Childhood: An Evolutionary-Developmental Synthesis." *Society for Research in Child Development*, November 10, 2014. https://doi.org/10.1111/cdep.12084

Kaplan, H., K. Hill, J. Lancaster, and A.M. Hurtado. "A Theory of Human Life History Evolution: Diet, Intelligence, and Longevity." *Evolutionary Anthropology*, August 16, 2000. https://doi.org/10.1002/1520-6505(2000)9:4<156::AID-EVAN5>3.0.CO;2-7

Penniman, L. *Farming While Black: Soul Fire Farm's Practical Guide to Liberation on the Land.* White River Junction, VT: Chelsea Green Publishing, 2018.

Walker, R., O. Burger, J. Wagner, and C.R. Von Rueden. "Evolution of Brain Size and Juvenile Periods in Primates." *Journal of Human Evolution*, July 5, 2006. https://doi.org/10.1016/j.jhevol.2006.06.002

Chapter 5: The Home Container

Barnes, J.D., and M.S. Tremblay. "Changes in Indicators of Child and Youth Physical Activity in Canada, 2005–2016." *Canadian Journal of Public Health*, November 1, 2016. https://doi.org/10.17269/CJPH.107.5645

Baykara, I., H. Yilmaz, T. Gültekin, and E. Güleç. "Squatting Facet: a Case Study Dilkaya and Van-Kalesi Populations in Eastern Turkey." *Collegium Antropologicum*, December 2010. https://pubmed.ncbi.nlm.nih.gov/21874707/

Berchicci, M., M.B. Pontifex, E.S. Drollette, C. Pesce, C.H. Hillman, and F. Di Russo. "From Cognitive Motor Preparation to Visual Processing: The Benefits of Childhood Fitness to Brain Health." *Neuroscience*, April 20, 2015. https://doi.org/10.1016/j.neuroscience.2015.04.028

Boulle, E.V. "Evolution of Two Human Skeletal Markers of the Squatting Position: A Diachronic Study from Antiquity to the Modern Age." *American Journal of Physical Anthropology*, April 12, 2001. https://doi.org/10.1002/ajpa.1055

Fain, E., and C. Weatherford. "Comparative Study of Millennials' (Age 20-34 Years) Grip and Lateral Pinch with the Norms." *Journal of Hand Therapy*, January 11, 2016. https://doi.org/10.1016/j.jht.2015.12.006

Grzybowski, A., P. Kanclerz, K. Tsubota, C. Lanca, and S.M. Saw . "A Review on the Epidemiology of Myopia in School Children Worldwide." *BMC Ophthalmology*, January 14, 2020. https://doi.org/10.1186/s12886-019-1220-0.

Katzenberg, M.A., and A.L. Grauer. *Biological Anthropology of the Human Skeleton*. Hoboken, NJ: John Wiley & Sons, 2019

Larson, L.R., R. Szczytko, E.P. Bowers, L.E. Stephens, K.T. Stevenson, and M.F. Floyd. "Outdoor Time, Screen Time, and Connection to Nature: Troubling Trends Among Rural Youth?" *Environment and Behavior*, October 1, 2019. https://doi.org/10.1177/0013916518806686

Oygucu, I. H., M. A. Kurt, I. Ikiz, T. Erem, and D. C. Davies. "Squatting Facets on the Neck of the Talus and Extensions of the Trochlear Surface of the Talus in Late Byzantine Males." *Journal of Anatomy*, December 18, 2002. https://doi.org/10.1046/j.1469-7580.1998.19220287.x

Peterson, M.D., P.M. Gordon, S. Smeding, and P. Visich. "Grip Strength Is Associated with Longitudinal Health Maintenance and Improvement in Adolescents." *The Journal of Pediatrics*, July 30, 2018. https://doi.org/10.1016/j.jpeds.2018.07.020

Raichlen, D.A., H. Pontzer, T.W. Zderic, J.A. Harris, A.Z.P. Mabulla, M.T. Hamilton, and B.M.

Wood. "Sitting, Squatting, and the Evolutionary Biology of Human Inactivity." *PNAS*. National Academy of Sciences, March 31, 2020. https://doi.org/10.1073/pnas.1911868117

Ramamurthy, D., S.Y. Lin Chua , and S.M Saw. "A Review of Environmental Risk Factors for Myopia during Early Life, Childhood and Adolescence." *Clinical & Experimental Optometry*, November 27, 2015. https://doi.org/10.1111/cxo.12346

Siddicky, S.F., J. Wang, B. Rabenhorst, L. Buchele, and E. M. Mannen. "Exploring Infant Hip Position and Muscle Activity in Common Baby Gear and Orthopedic Devices." *Journal of Orthopedic Research*, July 31, 2020. https://doi.org/10.1002/jor.24818

Townsend, J.B., and S. Barton. "The Impact of Ancient Tree Form on Modern Landscape Preferences." *Urban Forestry & Urban Greening*, June 18, 2018. https://doi.org/10.1016/j.ufug.2018.06.004

Chapter 6: The Learning Container

America Walks. "How to Conduct a Walk Audit in Your Community – Quick Video Guide for Assessing Your Neighborhood Walkability." *AmericaWalks*. Accessed 2021. https://americawalks.org/how-to-conduct-a-walk-audit-in-your-community-quick-guide-for-assessing-your-neighborhood-walkability/

Arundell, L., J. Salmon, H. Koorts, A. Ayala, and A. Timperio. "Exploring When and How Adolescents Sit: Cross-Sectional Analysis of ActivPAL-Measured Patterns of Daily Sitting Time, Bouts and Breaks." BMC Public Health. BioMed Central, June 11, 2019. https://doi.org/10.1186/s12889-019-6960-5

Baepler, P., J.D. Walker, and M. Driessen. "It's Not about Seat Time: Blending, Flipping, and Efficiency in Active Learning Classrooms." *Computers & Education*. Pergamon, June 18, 2014. https://doi.org/10.1016/j.compedu.2014.06.006

Griffiths, L., M. Cortina-Borja, and F. Sera. "How Active Are Our Children? Findings from the Millennium Cohort Study." *BMJ Open*, August 21, 2013. https://doi.org/10.1136/bmjopen-2013-002893

Jago, R., R. Salway, L. Emm-Collison, S. Sebire, J. Thompson, and D. Lawlor. "Association of BMI Category with Change in Children's Physical Activity between Ages 6 and 11 Years: a Longitudinal Study." *International Journal of Obesity*, November 12, 2019. https://doi.org/10.1038/s41366-019-0459-0

Kahan, D. "Recess, Extracurricular Activities, and Active Classrooms." *Journal of Physical Education, Recreation & Dance,* January 26, 2013. https://doi.org/10.1080/07303084.2008.10598131

Martin, R., and E.M. Murtagh. "Teachers' and Students' Perspectives of Participating in the 'Active Classrooms' Movement Integration Programme." *Teaching and Teacher Education.* Pergamon, January 13, 2017. https://doi.org/10.1016/j.tate.2017.01.002

Prater, M., A. Jenkins, and C. Mulrine. "The Active Classroom: Supporting Students with Attention Deficit Hyperactivity Disorder through Exercise." *TEACHING Exceptional Children,* May 1, 2008. https://doi.org/10.1177/004005990804000502

Ridgers, N., A. Timperio, D. Crawford, and J. Salmon. "Five-Year Changes in School Recess and Lunchtime and the Contribution to Children's Daily Physical Activity." *British Journal of Sports Medicine.* BMJ Publishing Group Ltd and British Association of Sport and Exercise Medicine, August 6, 2012. http://dx.doi.org/10.1136/bjsm.2011.084921

Rollo, S., L. Crutchlow, T. Nagpal, W. Sui , and H. Prapavessis. "The Effects of Classroom-Based Dynamic Seating Interventions on Academic Outcomes in Youth: a Systematic Review." *Learning Environments Research*, August 10, 2018. https://doi.org/https://doi.org/10.1007/s10984-018-9271-3

Safe Routes to School National Partnership. "Get to Know Your Neighborhood With a Walk Audit." *Safe Routes Partnership*, 2018. https://www.saferoutespartnership.org/resources/fact-sheet/walk-audit-factsheet

Walmsley, N., and D. Westall. *Forest School Adventure: Outdoor Skills and Play for Children.* East Sussex: Guild of Master Craftsman Publications, 2018.

Walmsley, N. *Urban Forest School: Outdoor Adventures and Skills for City Kids.* East Sussex, UK: Guild of Master Craftsman Publications, Ltd, 2020.

Chapter 7: The Activities Container

Fuchs, R.K., J.J. Bauer, and C.M. Snow. "Jumping Improves Hip and Lumbar Spine Bone Mass in Prepubescent Children: a Randomized Controlled Trial." *Journal of Bone and Mineral Research*, January 16, 2001. https://doi.org/10.1359/jbmr.2001.16.1.148

Hightower, L. "Osteoporosis: Pediatric Disease with Geriatric Consequences." *Orthopaedic Nursing,* 2000. https://doi.org/10.1097/00006416-200019050-00010

Larson, L.R., GT. Green, and H.K. Cordell. "Children's Time Outdoors: Results and Implications of the National Kids Survey." *Journal of Park and Recreation Administration,* 2011. https://doi.org/10.1093/pubmed/fdy071

Lin, S.J., and S.C. Yang. "The Development of Fundamental Movement Skills by Children Aged Six to Nine." *Universal Journal of Educational Research*, 2015. https://doi.org/10.13189/ujer.2015.031211

Lubans, D.R., P.J. Morgan, D.P. Cliff, L.M. Barnett, and A.D. Okely. "Fundamental Movement Skills in Children and Adolescents." *Sports Medicine*, September 23, 2012. https://doi.org/10.2165/11536850-000000000-00000

Mirtz, T.A., J.P. Chandler, and C.M. Eyers. "The Effects of Physical Activity on the Epiphyseal Growth Plates: a Review of the Literature on Normal Physiology and Clinical Implications." *Journal of Clinical Medicine Research,* February 12, 2011. https://doi.org/10.4021/jocmr477w

Weaver, C.M., C.M. Gordon, K.F. Janz, H.J. Kalkwarf, J.M. Lappe, R. Lewis, M. O'Karma, T.C. Wallace, and B.S. Zemel. "The National Osteoporosis Foundation's Position Statement on Peak Bone Mass Development and Lifestyle Factors: a Systematic Review and Implementation Recommendations." *Osteoporosis International,* February 8, 2016. https://doi.org/10.1007/s00198-015-3440-3

Chapter 9: Alloparents

Kenkel, W.M., A.M. Perkeybile, and C.S. Carter. "The Neurobiological Causes and Effects of Alloparenting." *Developmental Neurobiology*, November 25, 2016. https://doi.org/10.1002/dneu.22465

Nadasdy, P. "First Nations, Citizenship and Animals, or Why Northern Indigenous People Might Not Want to Live in Zoopolis: Canadian Journal of Political Science/Revue Canadienne De Science Politique." *Canadian Journal of Political Science.* February 5, 2016. https://doi.org/10.1017/S0008423915001079

Page, A.E., M.G. Thomas, D. Smith, M. Dyble, S. Viguier, N. Chaudhary, G.D. Salali, J. Thompson, R. Mace, and A.B. Migliano. "Testing Adaptive Hypotheses of Alloparenting in Agta Foragers." *Nature Human Behaviour*, August 12, 2019. https://doi.org/10.1038/s41562-019-0679-2

Riedman, M.L. "The Evolution of Alloparental Care and Adoption in Mammals and Birds." *The Quarterly Review of Biology,* December 4, 1982. https://doi.org/10.1086/412936

Solomon, A. *Far from the Tree: Parents, Children and the Search for Identity*. New York, NY: Scribner, 2014.

Volk, A.A. "Human Breastfeeding Is Not Automatic." *Journal of Social, Evolutionary, and Cultural Psychology,* 2009. http://dx.doi.org/10.1037/h0099314

Afterword

Dunton, G.F., B. Do, and S.D. Wang. "Early Effects of the COVID-19 Pandemic on Physical Activity and Sedentary Behavior in Children Living in the U.S." *BMC Public Health*. BioMed Central, September 4, 2020. https://doi.org/10.1186/s12889-020-09429-3

Howard, C.R., and N.F. Fletcher. "Emerging Virus Diseases: Can We Ever Expect the Un-expected?" *Emerging Microbes & Infections*, December 26, 2012. http://doi.org/10.1038/emi.2012.47

Keusch, G., M. Pappaioanou, and M.C. Gonzalez. "Drivers of Zoonotic Diseases." *Sustaining Global Surveillance and Response to Emerging Zoonotic Diseases*. Washington, DC: National Academies Press, 2009.

O'Dowd, A. "Infectious Diseases Are Spreading More Rapidly than Ever before, WHO Warns." *The BMJ*, August 30, 2007. http://doi.org/10.1136/bmj.39318.516968.DB

U.S. Department of Labor. "List of Goods Produced by Child Labor or Forced Labor." Accessed 2021. dol.gov/sites/dolgov/files/ILAB/child_labor_reports/tda2019/2020_TVPRA_List_Online_Final.pdf

PHOTO CREDITS

All photos from Katy Bowman except:

INDEX